As Proud as a Peacock

Illustrated
English Sayings

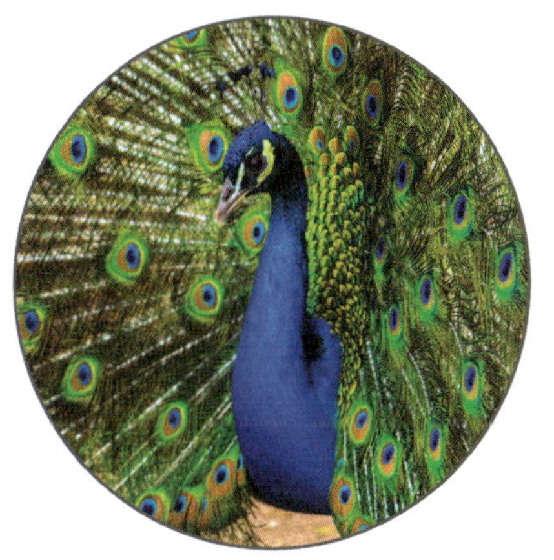

This book belongs to

There are four sections in this book

- Animal kingdom
- Precious things
- World of nature
- Strange expressions

Each section starts with a quiz, like this...

As proud as a _ _ _ _ _ _ _ .

TIP: The 7 dashes show this missing word has 7 letters.

Keep reading to check your answers. You may sometimes know a different answer!

Quick Quiz 1
Animal kingdom

1 **As proud as a _ _ _ _ _ _ _ _ .**

2 **As brave as a _ _ _ _ _ .**

3 **As cunning as a _ _ _ _ .**

4 **As busy as a _ _ _ .**

5 **As gentle as a _ _ _ _ .**

6 **As strong as an _ _ .**

7 **As wise as an _ _ _ .**

Answers coming up!

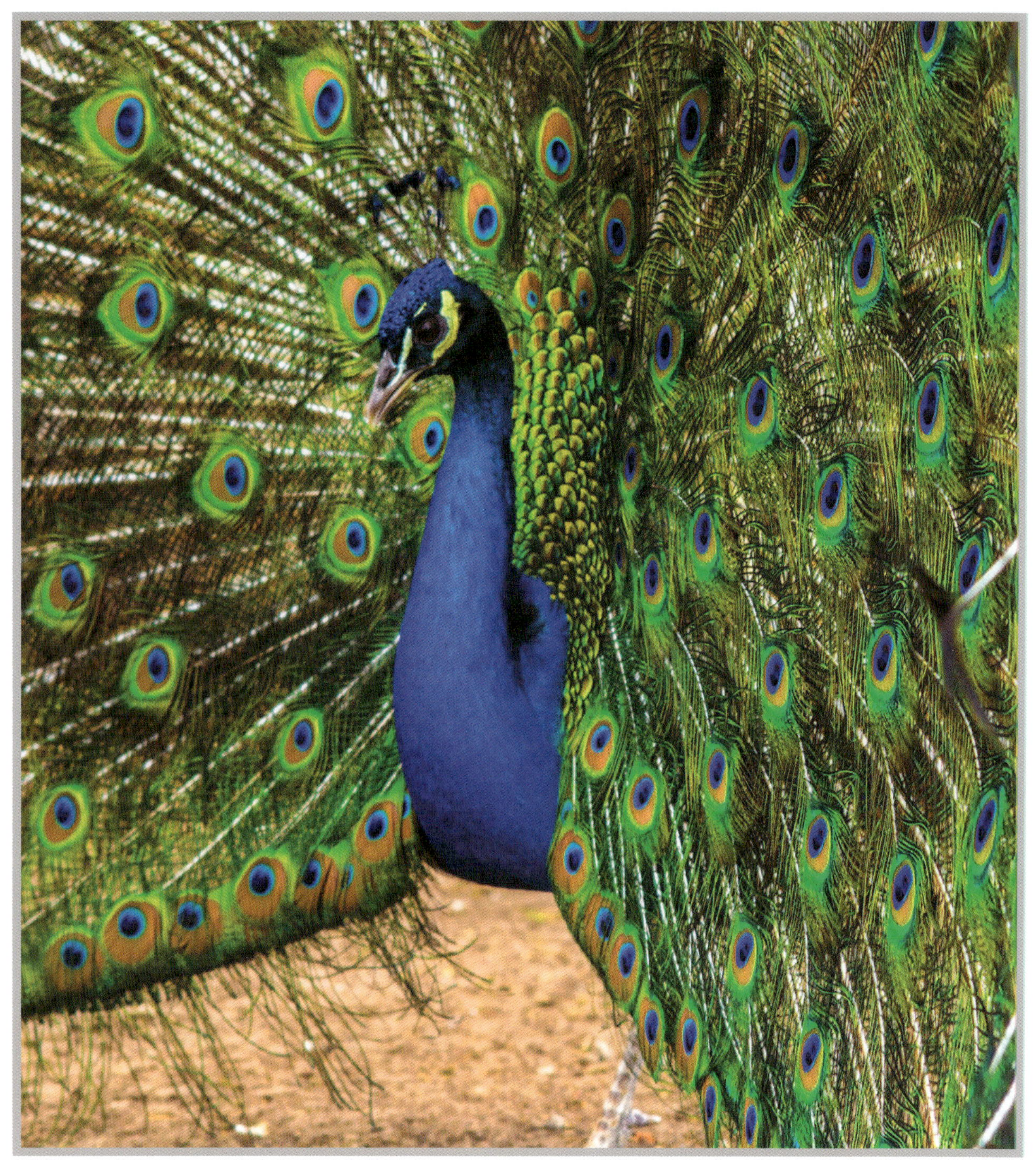

As proud as a peacock.

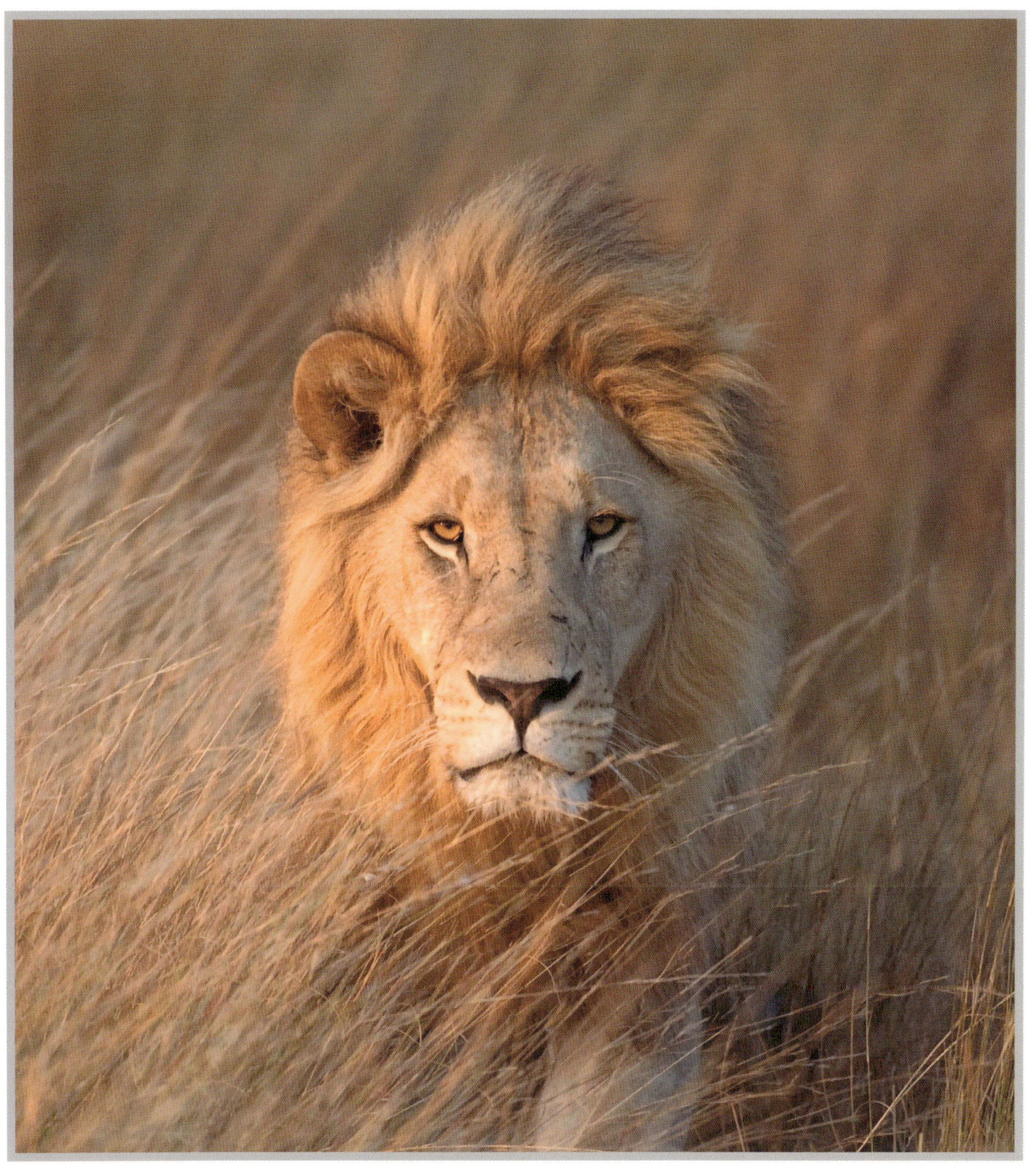

As brave as a lion.

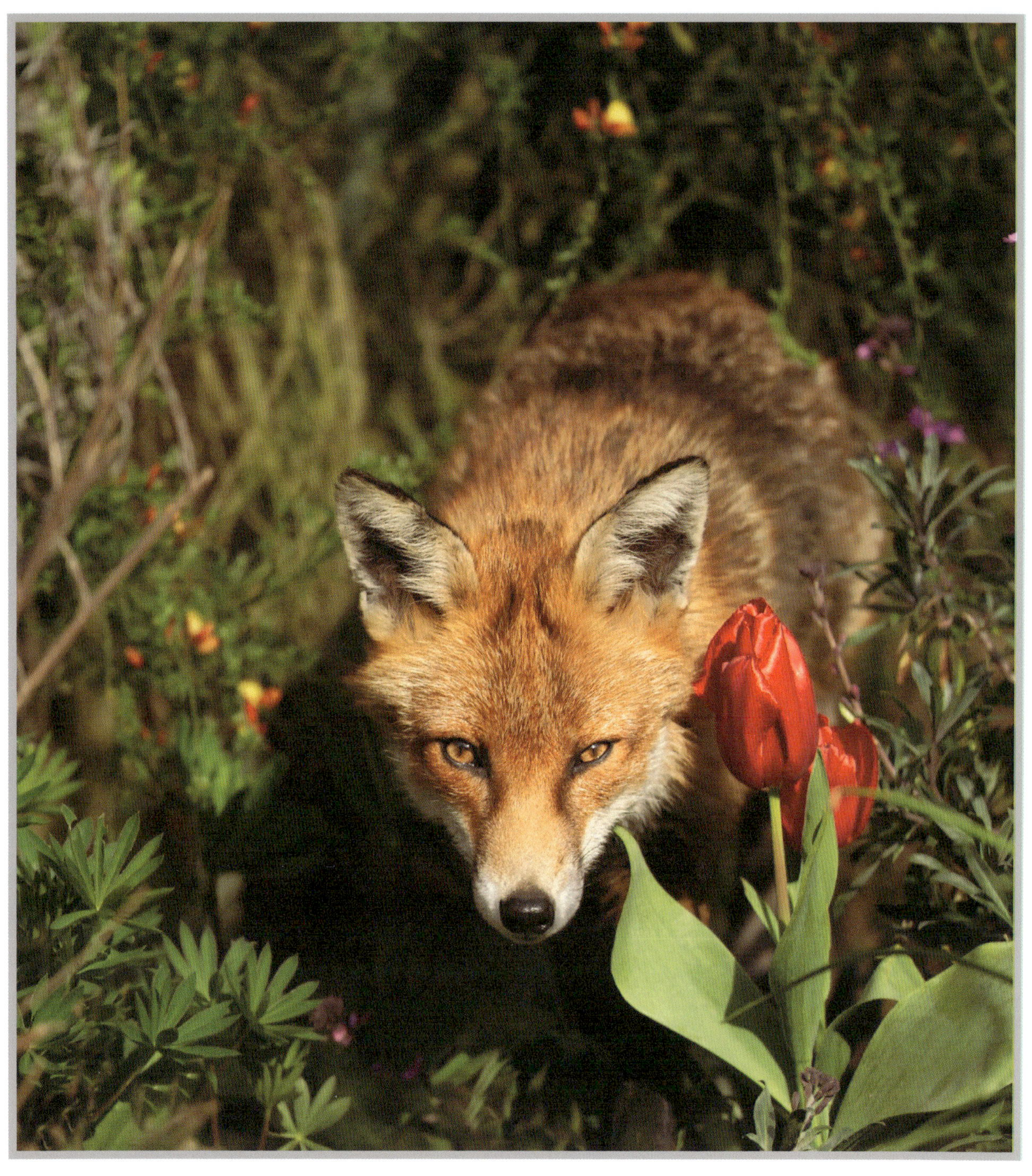

As cunning as a fox.

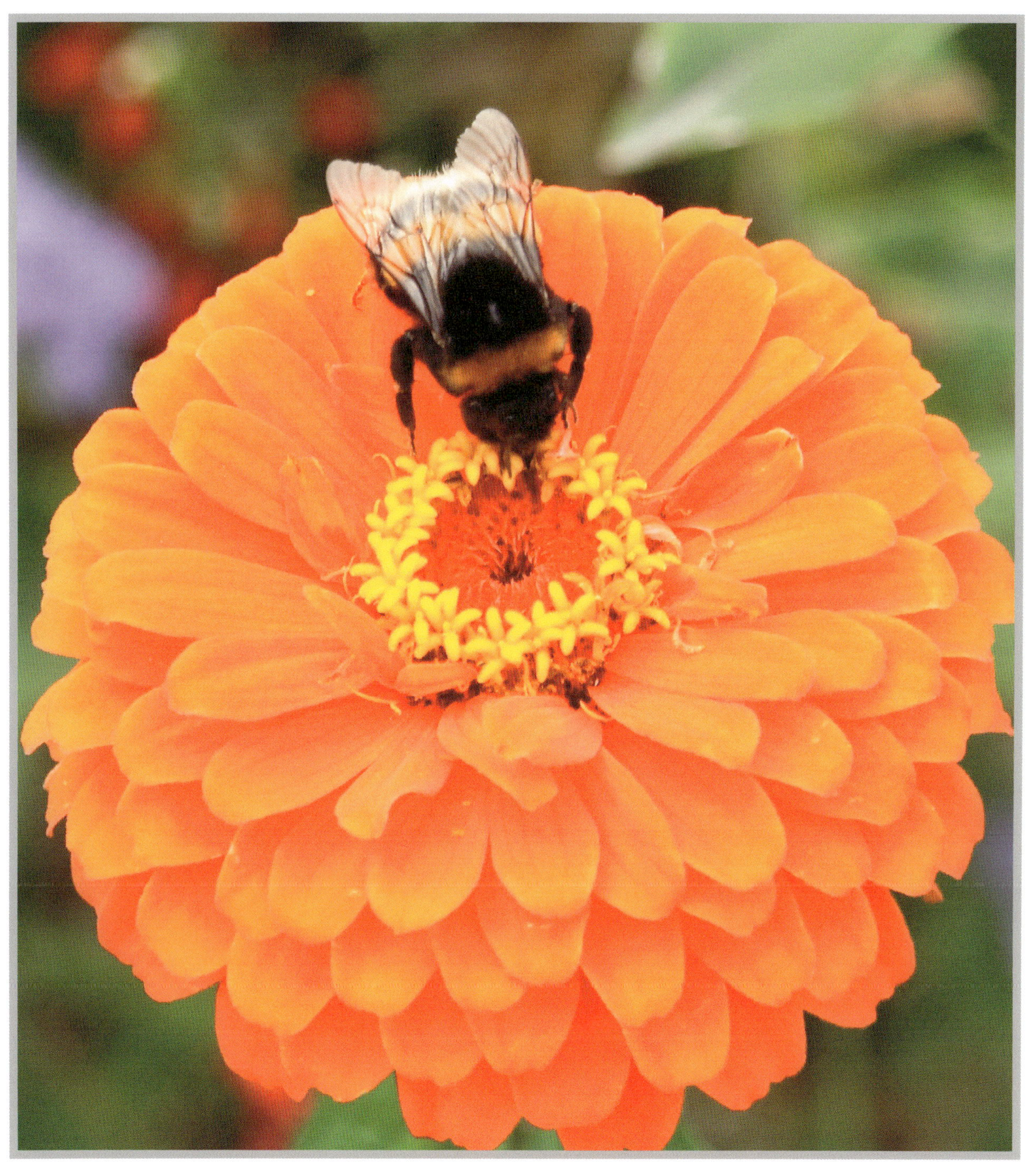

As busy as a bee.

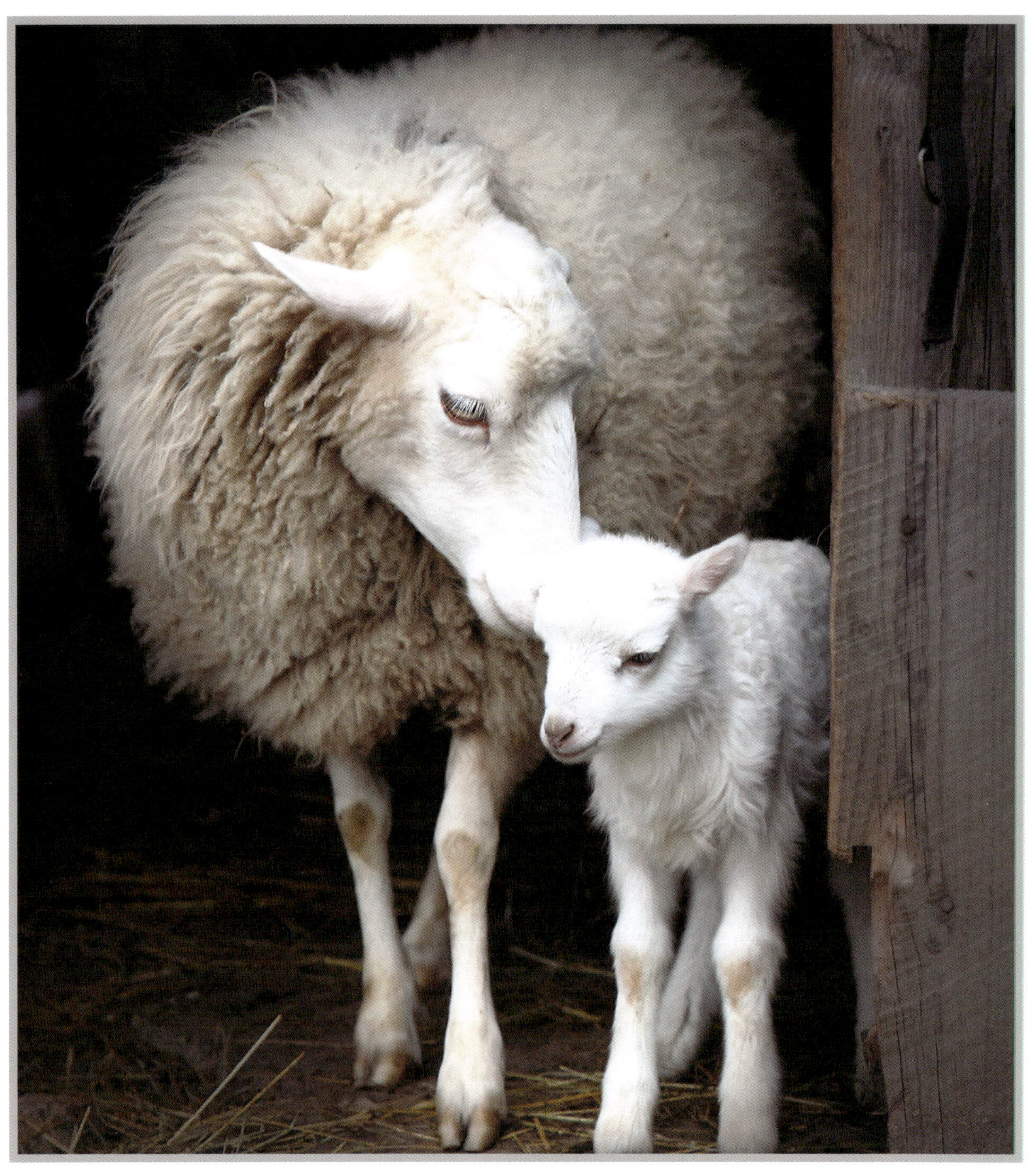

As gentle as a lamb.

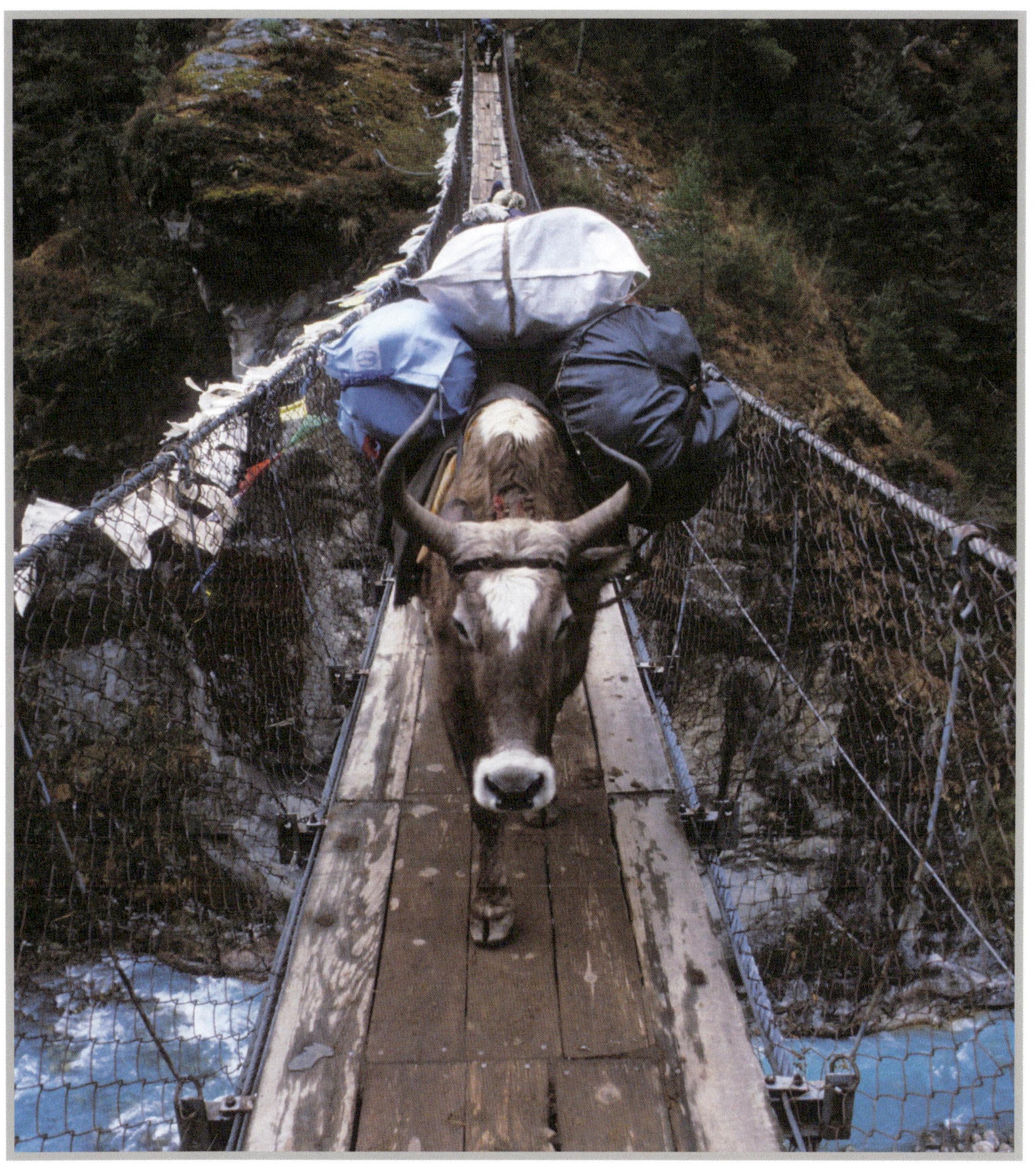

As strong as an ox.

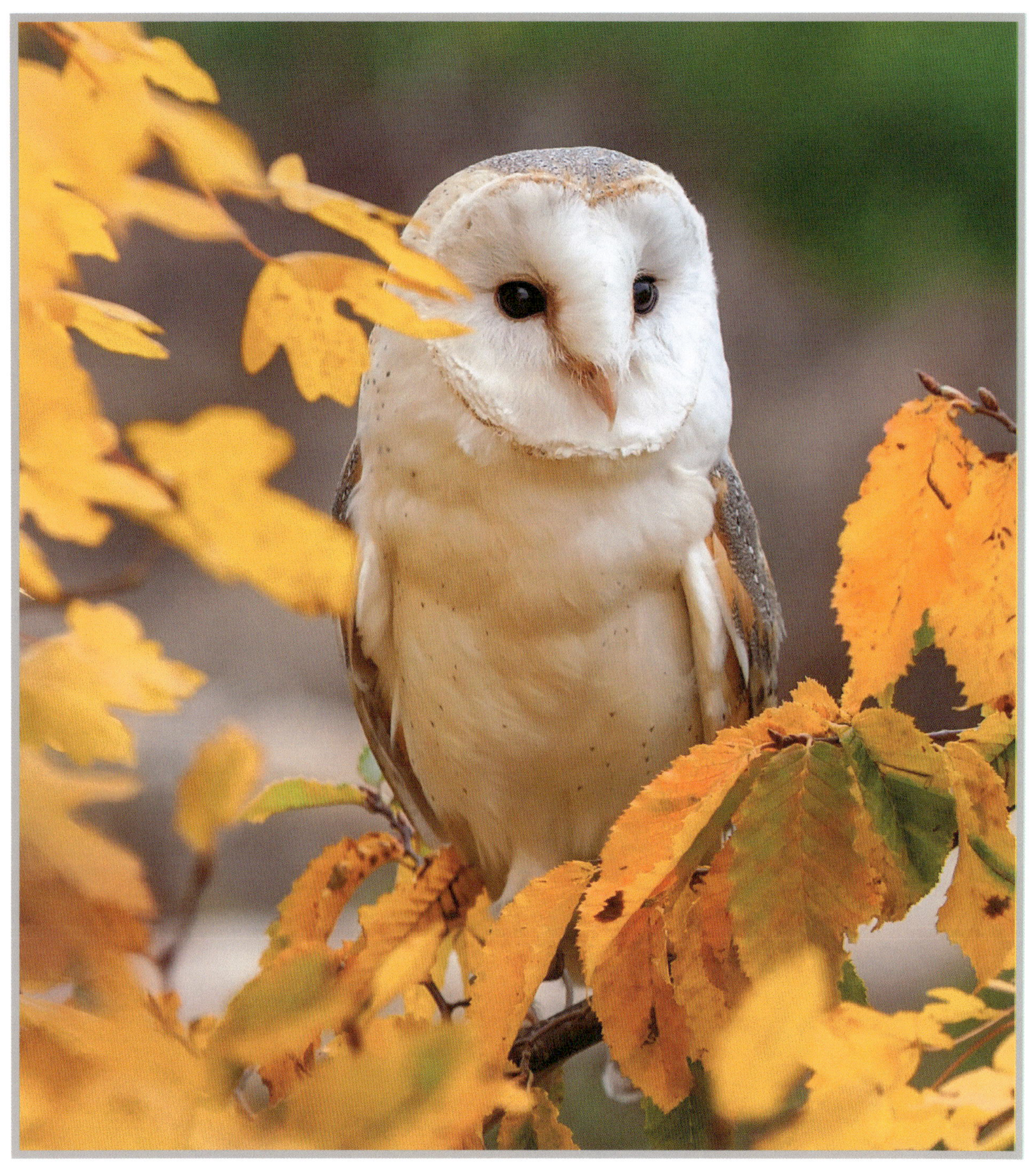

As wise as an owl.

Quick Quiz 2:
Precious things

1 **As soft as** _ _ _ _ _ _ .

2 **As clear as** _ _ _ _ _ _ _ .

3 **As smooth as** _ _ _ _ .

4 **As good as** _ _ _ _ .

5 **As bold as** _ _ _ _ _ .

6 **As still as a** _ _ _ _ _ _ .

7 **As pretty as a** _ _ _ _ _ _ _ .

Answers coming up!

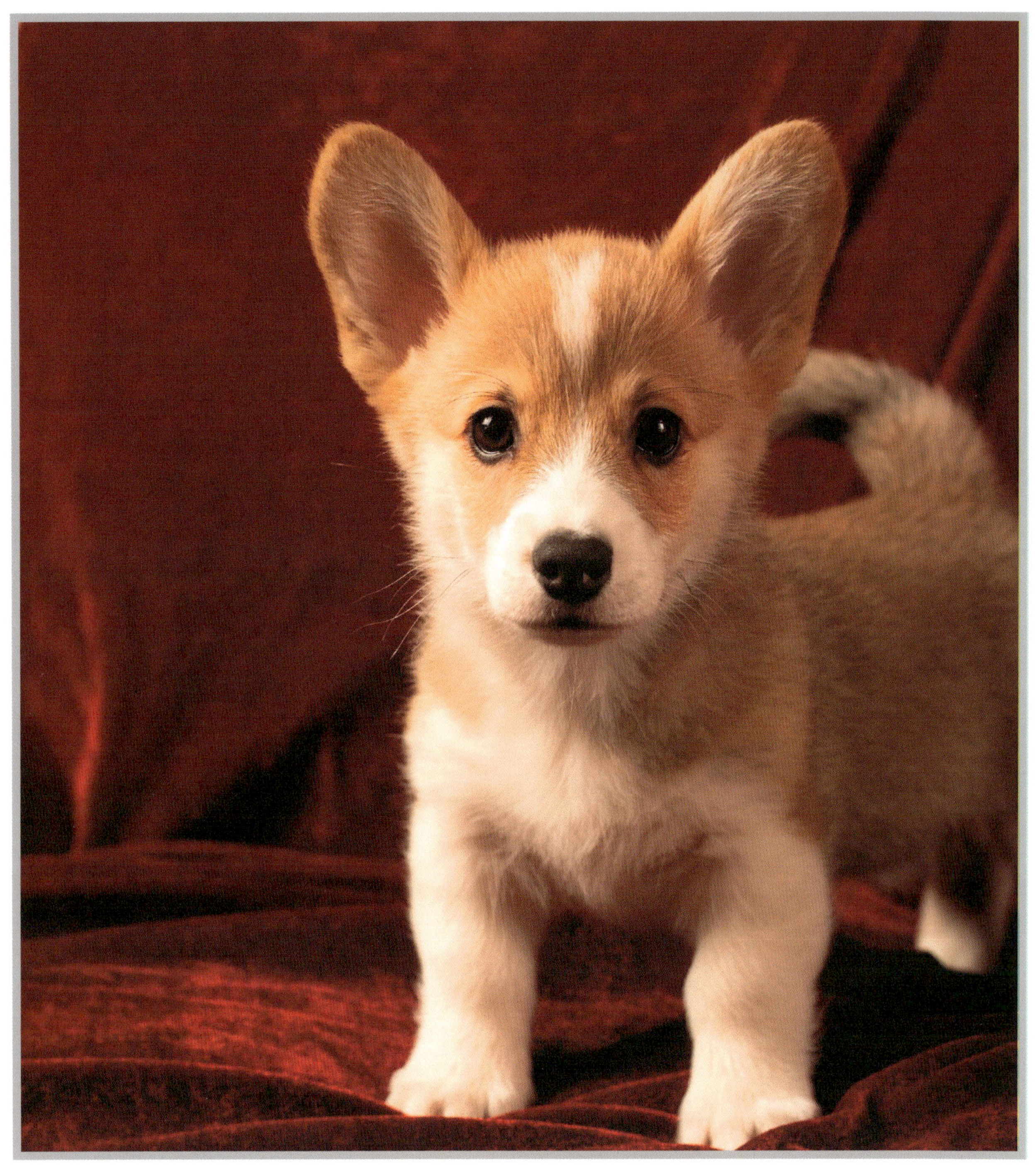

As soft as velvet.

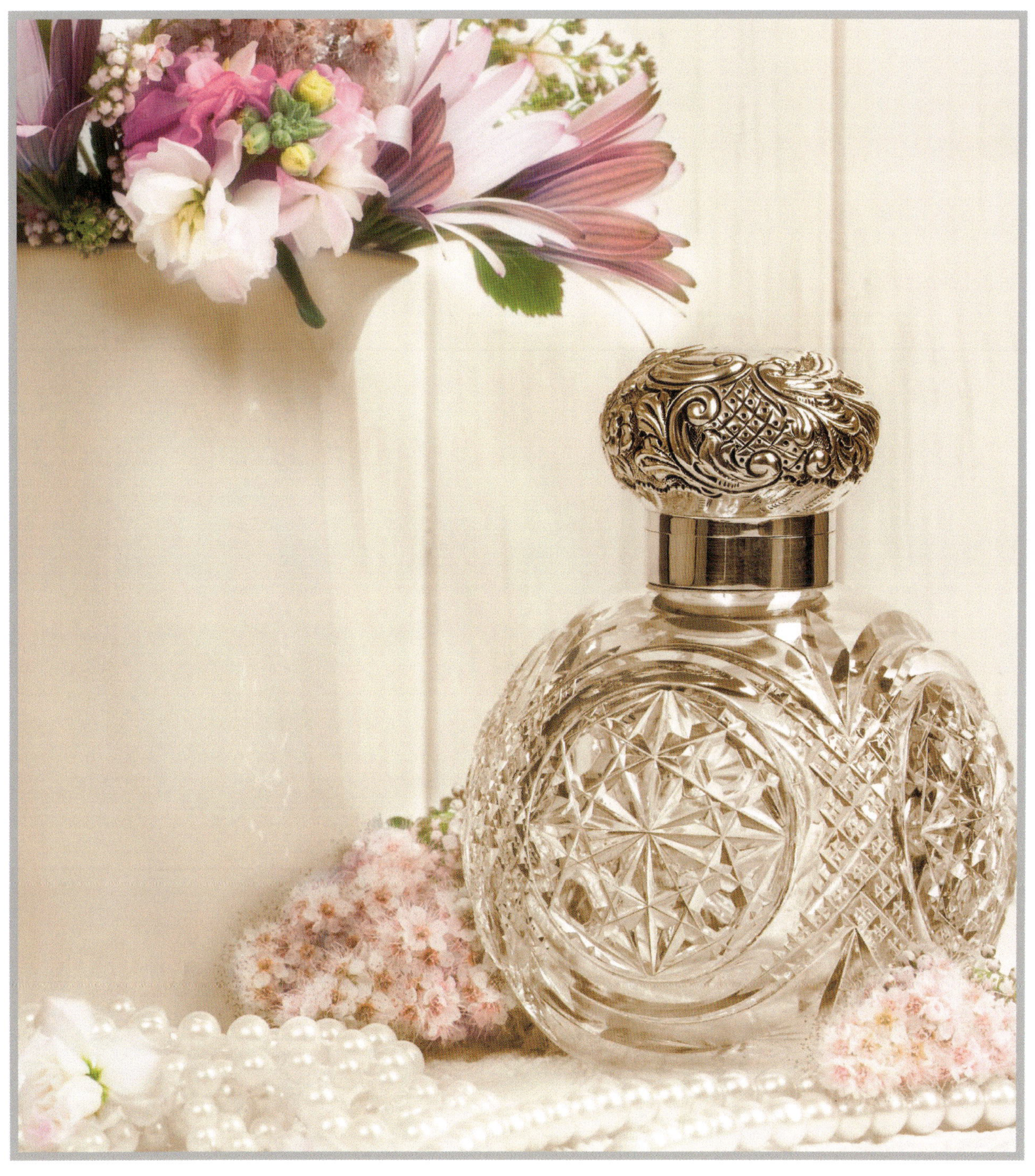

As clear as crystal.

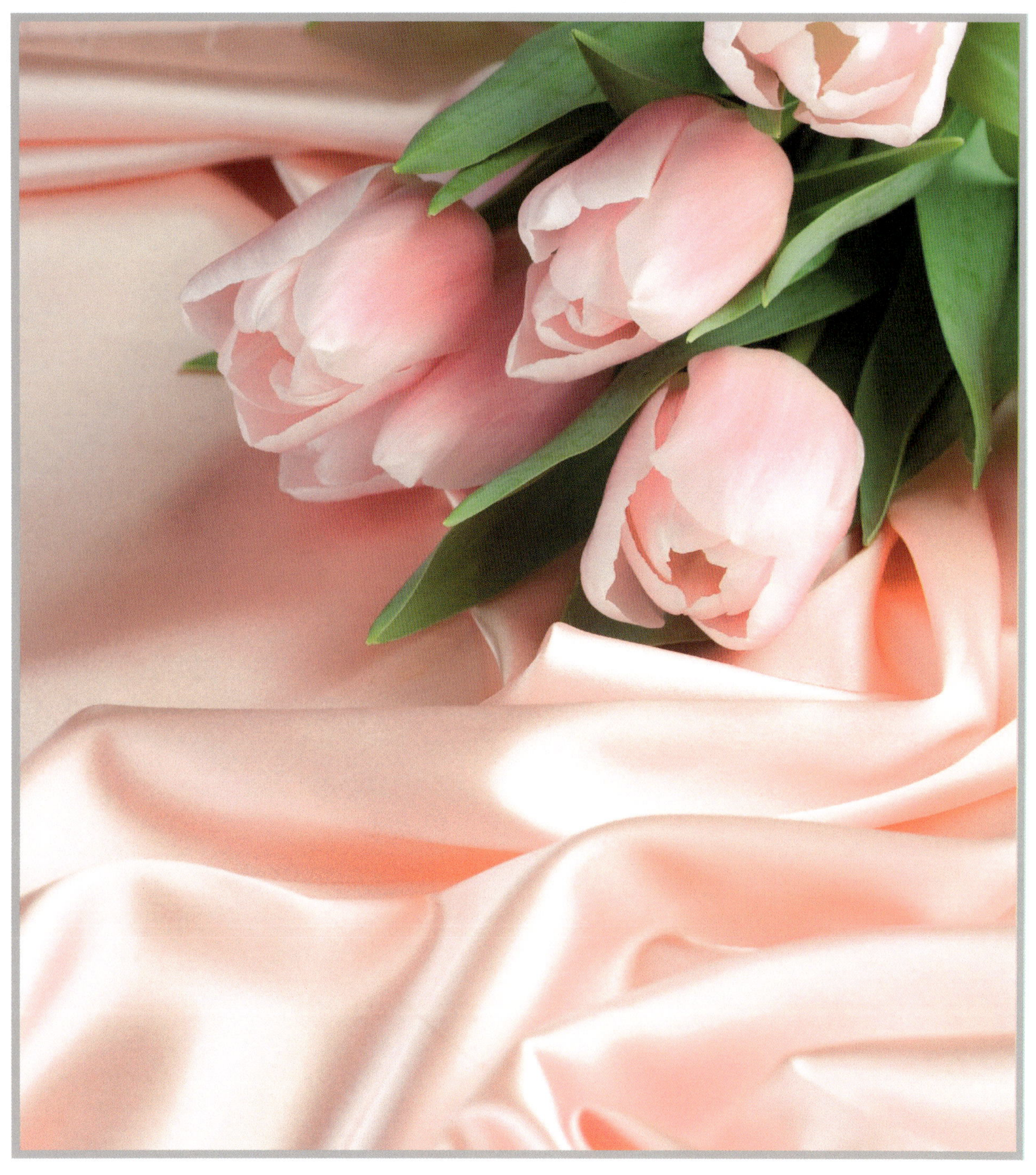

As smooth as silk.

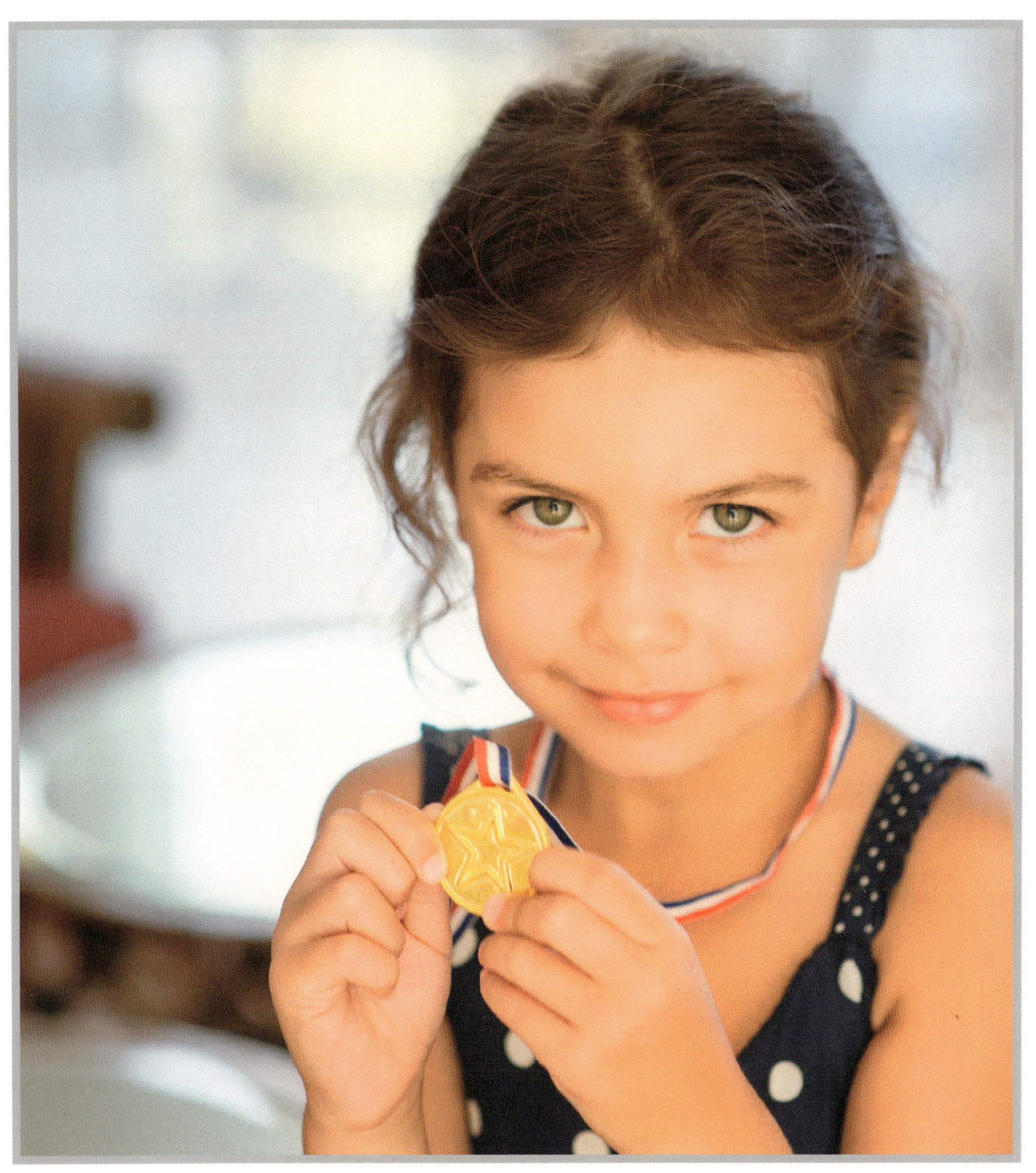

As good as gold.

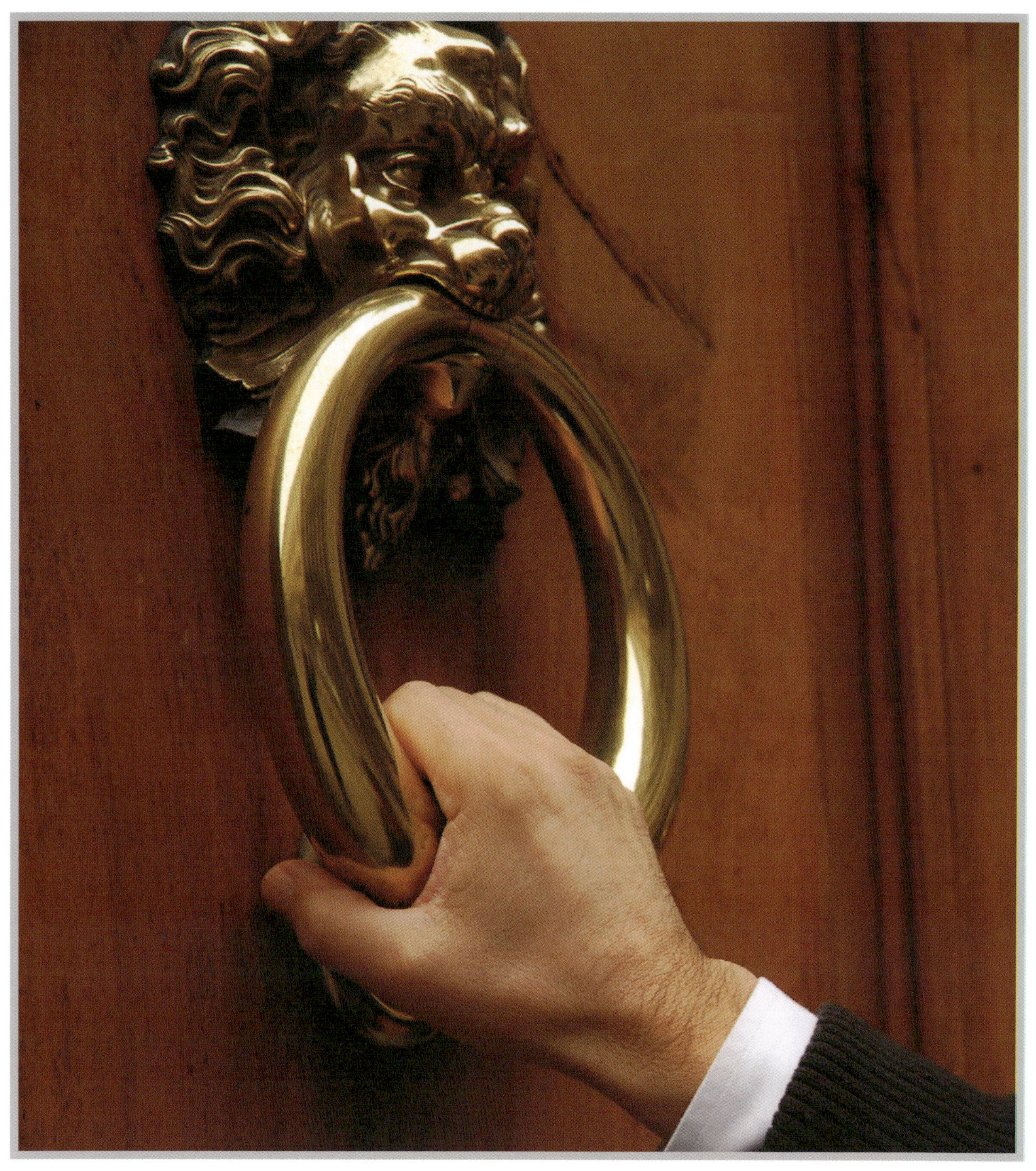

As bold as brass.

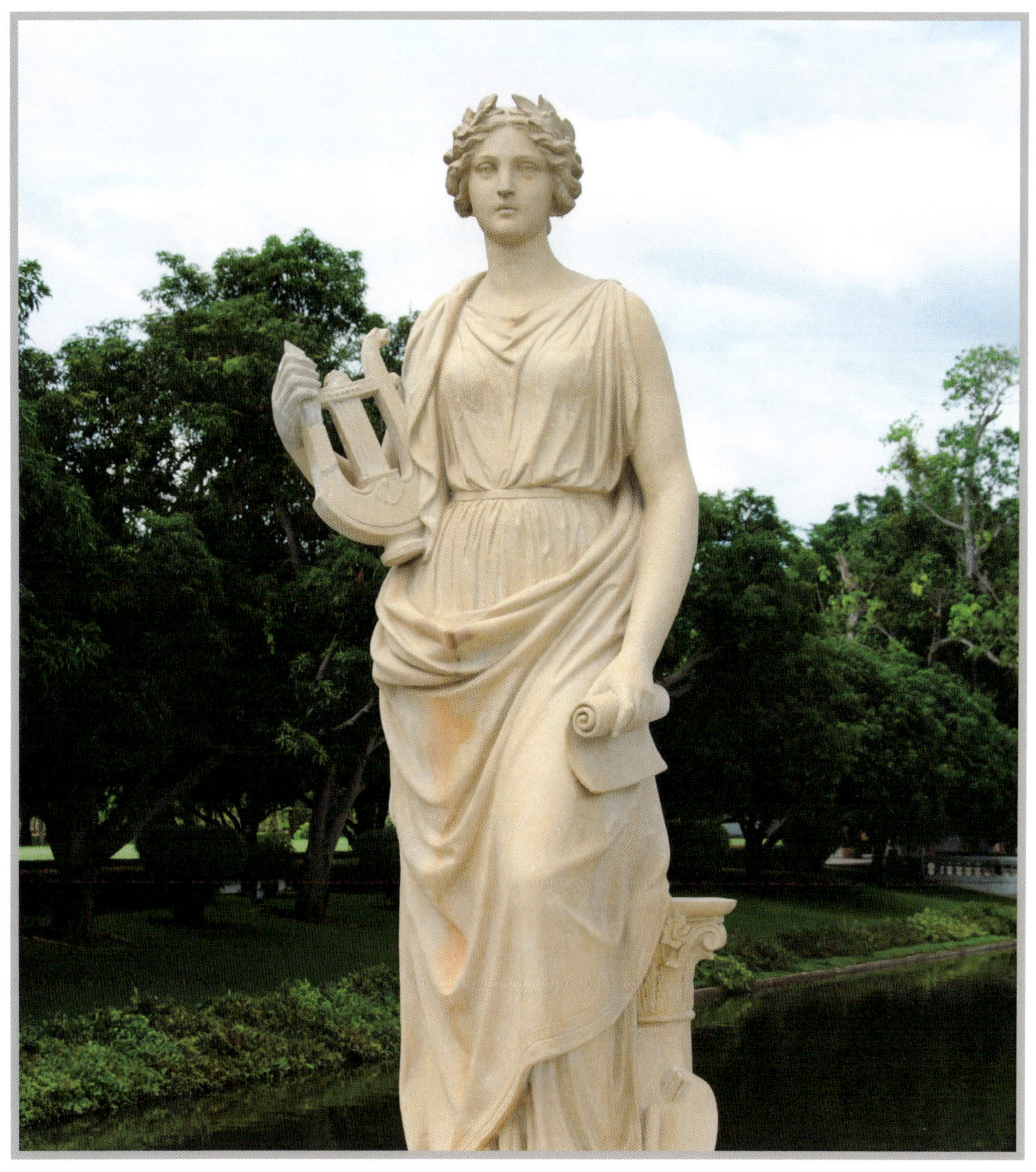

As still as a statue.

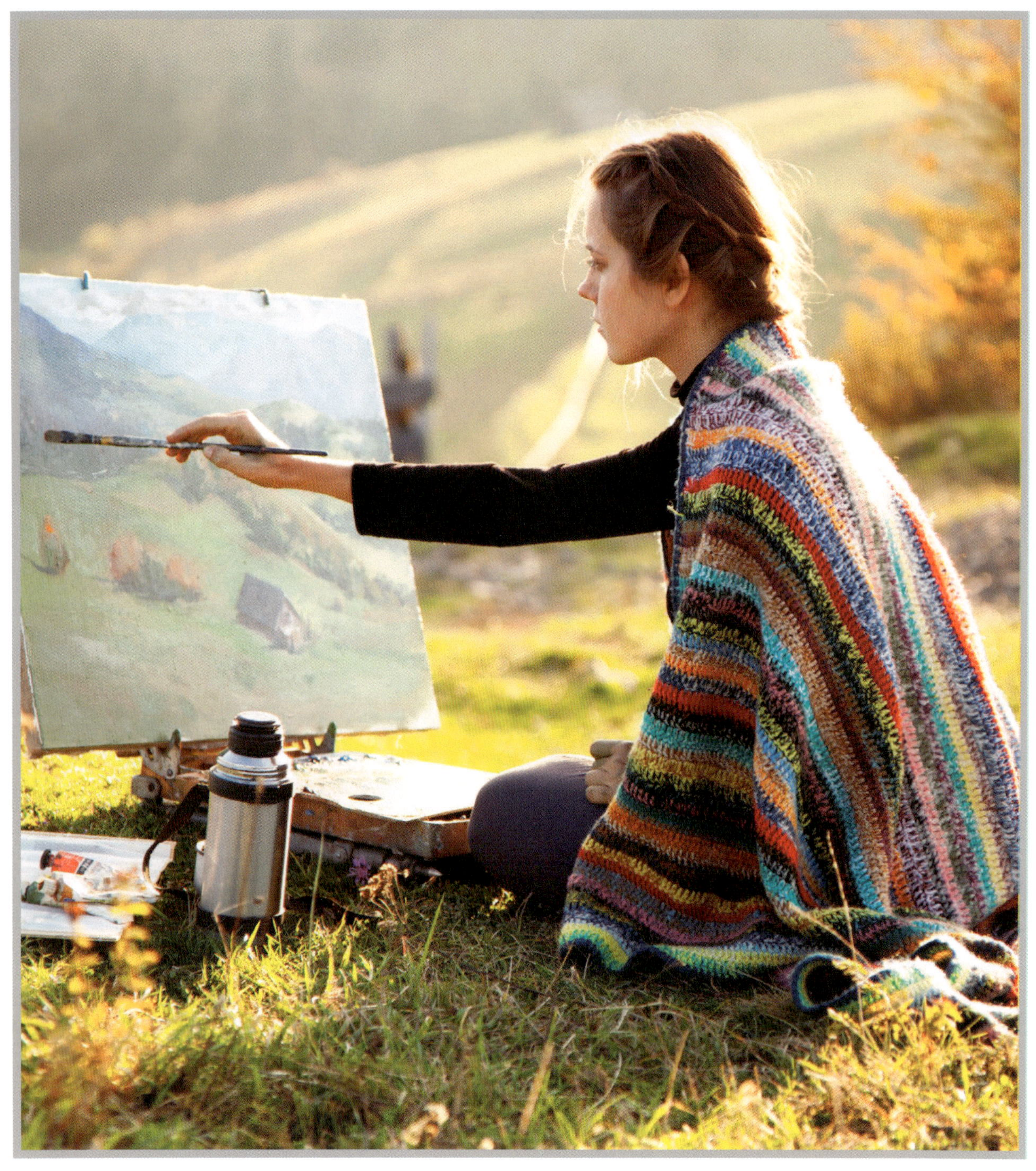

As pretty as a picture.

Quick Quiz 3:
World of nature

1 As cold as _ _ _ .

2 As pure as the driven _ _ _ _ _ .

3 As green as _ _ _ _ _ _ .

4 As solid as a _ _ _ _ _ .

5 As old as the _ _ _ _ _ _ .

6 As calm as a _ _ _ _ _ _ _ _ _ .

7 As deep as the _ _ _ _ _ _ .

Answers coming up!

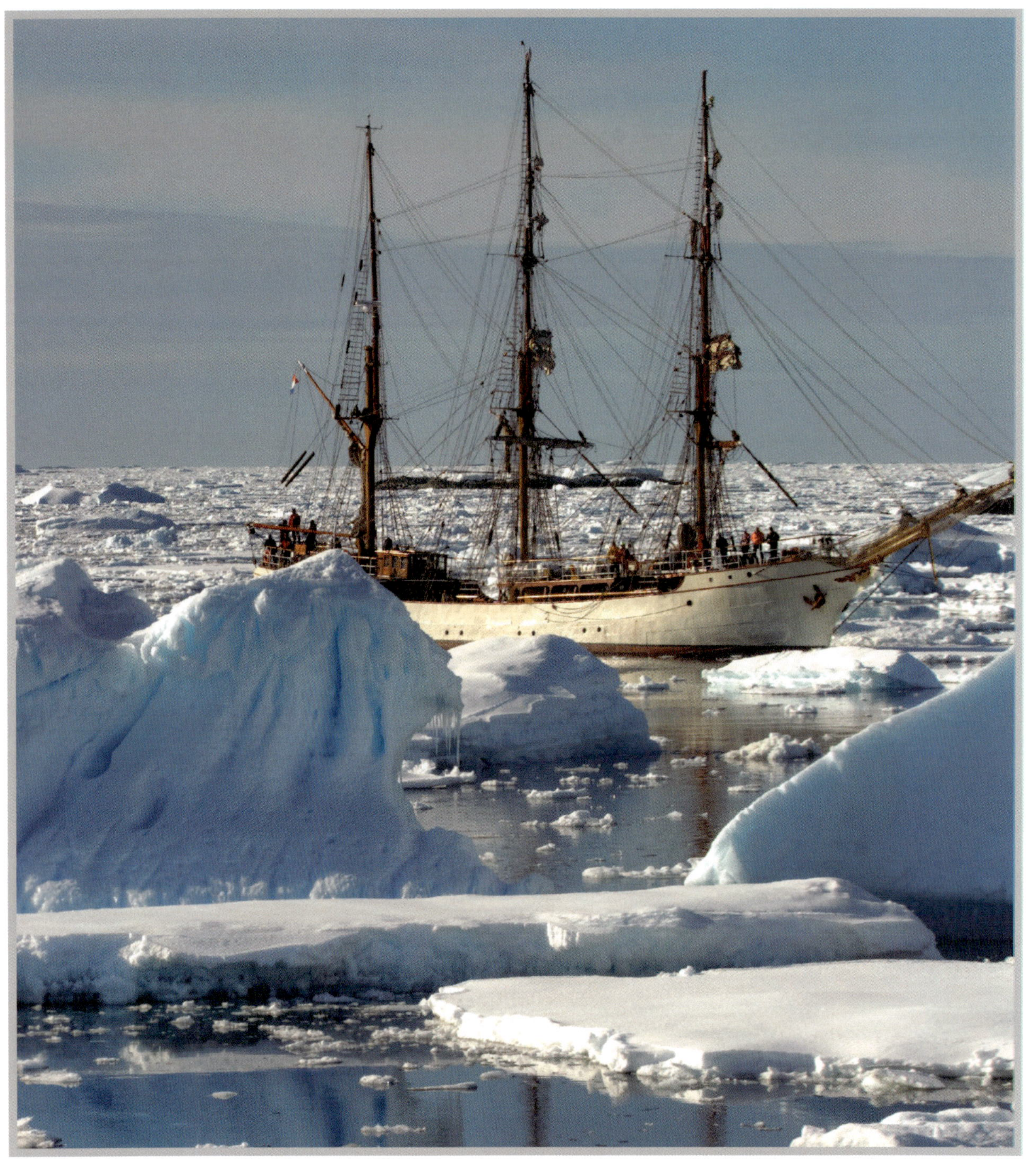

As cold as ice.

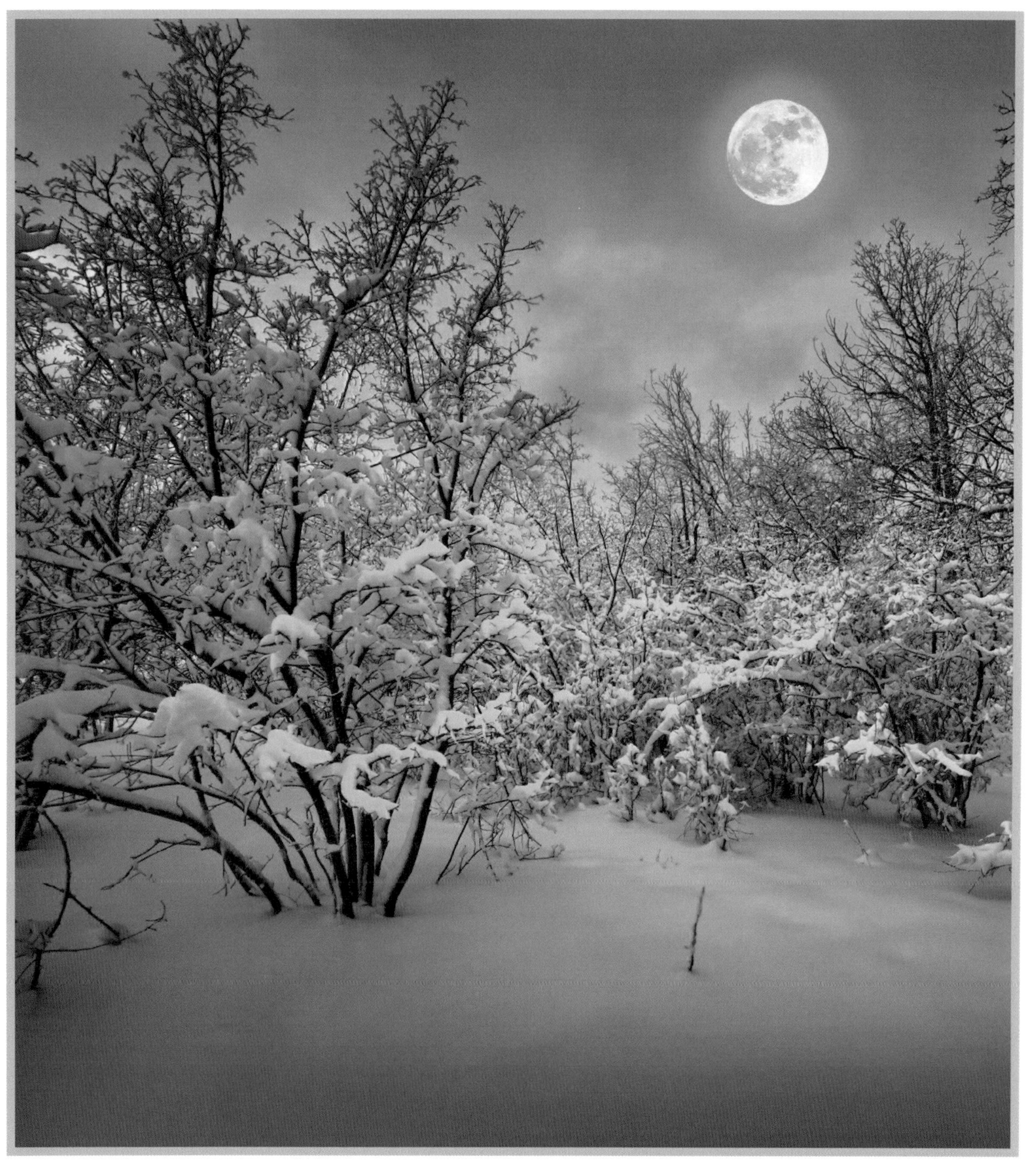

As pure as the driven snow.

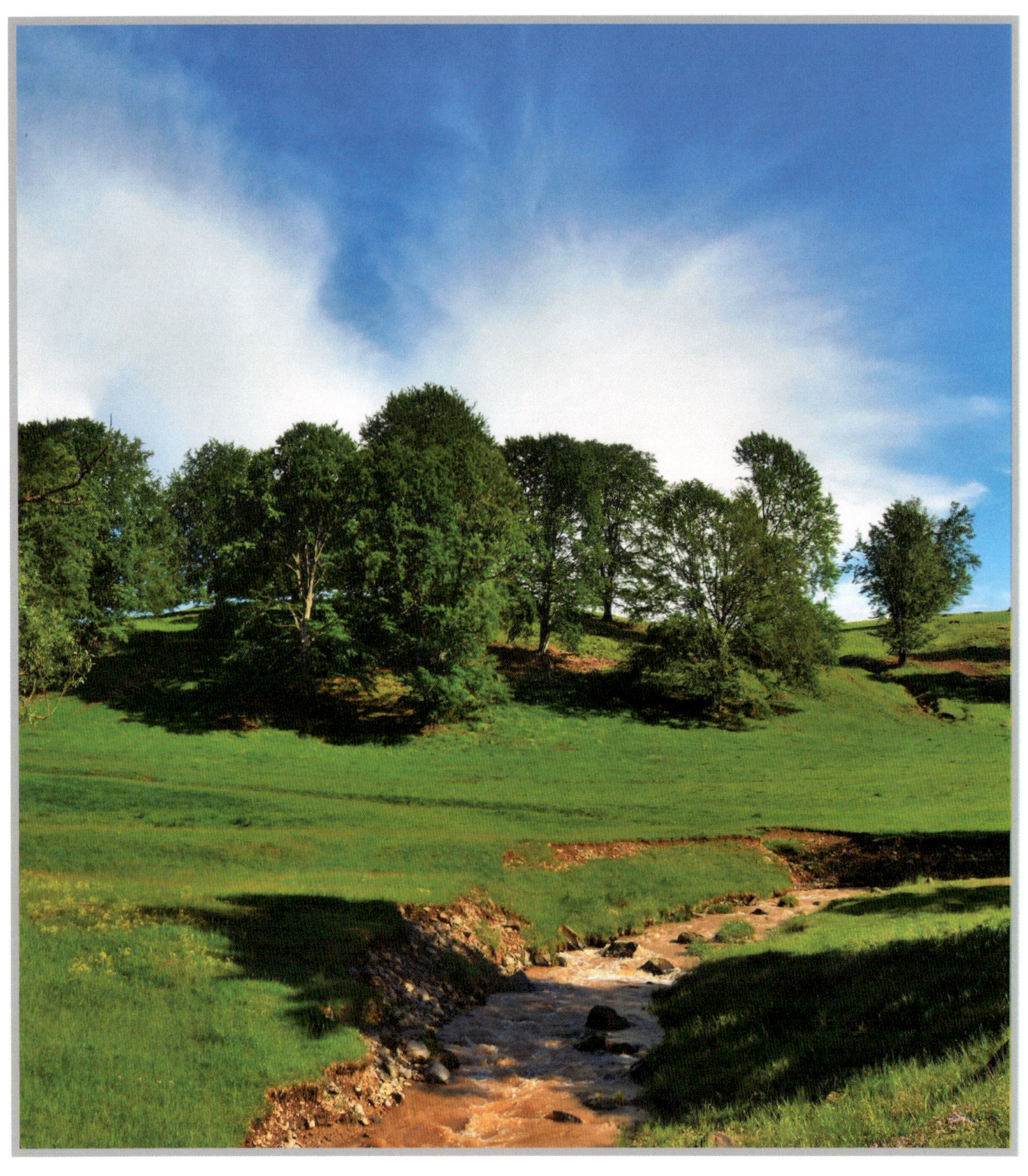

As green as grass.

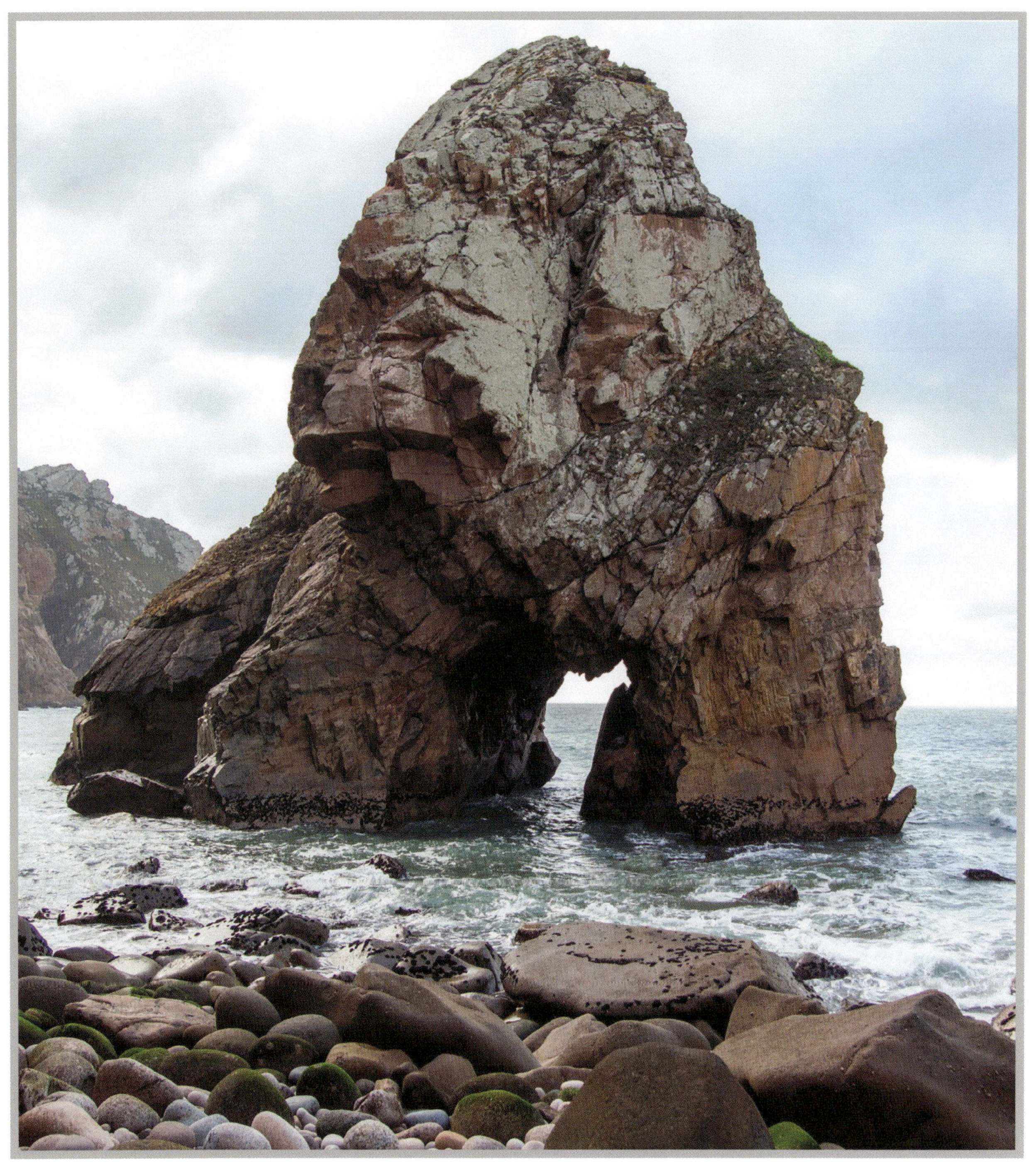

As solid as a rock.

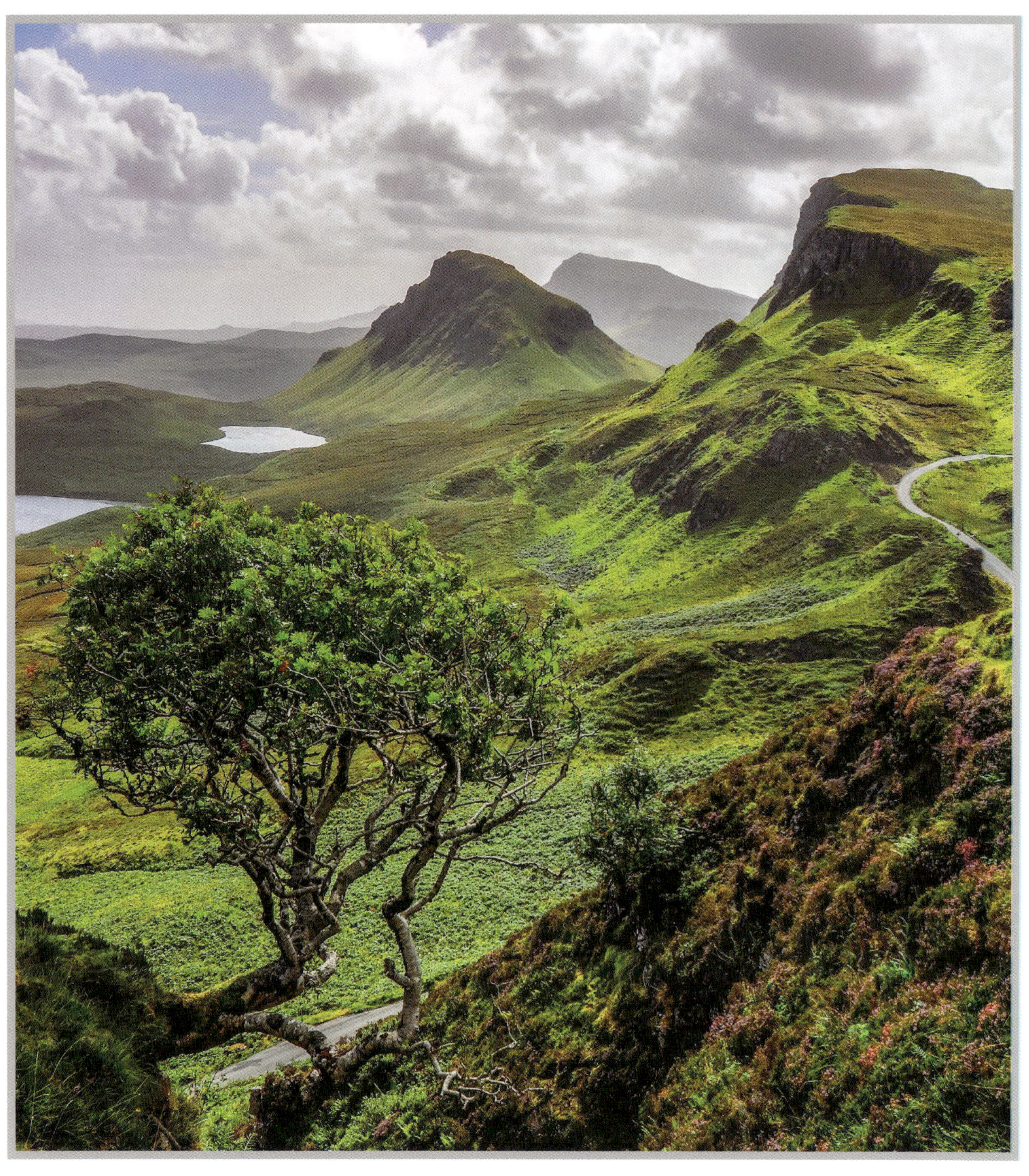

As old as the hills.

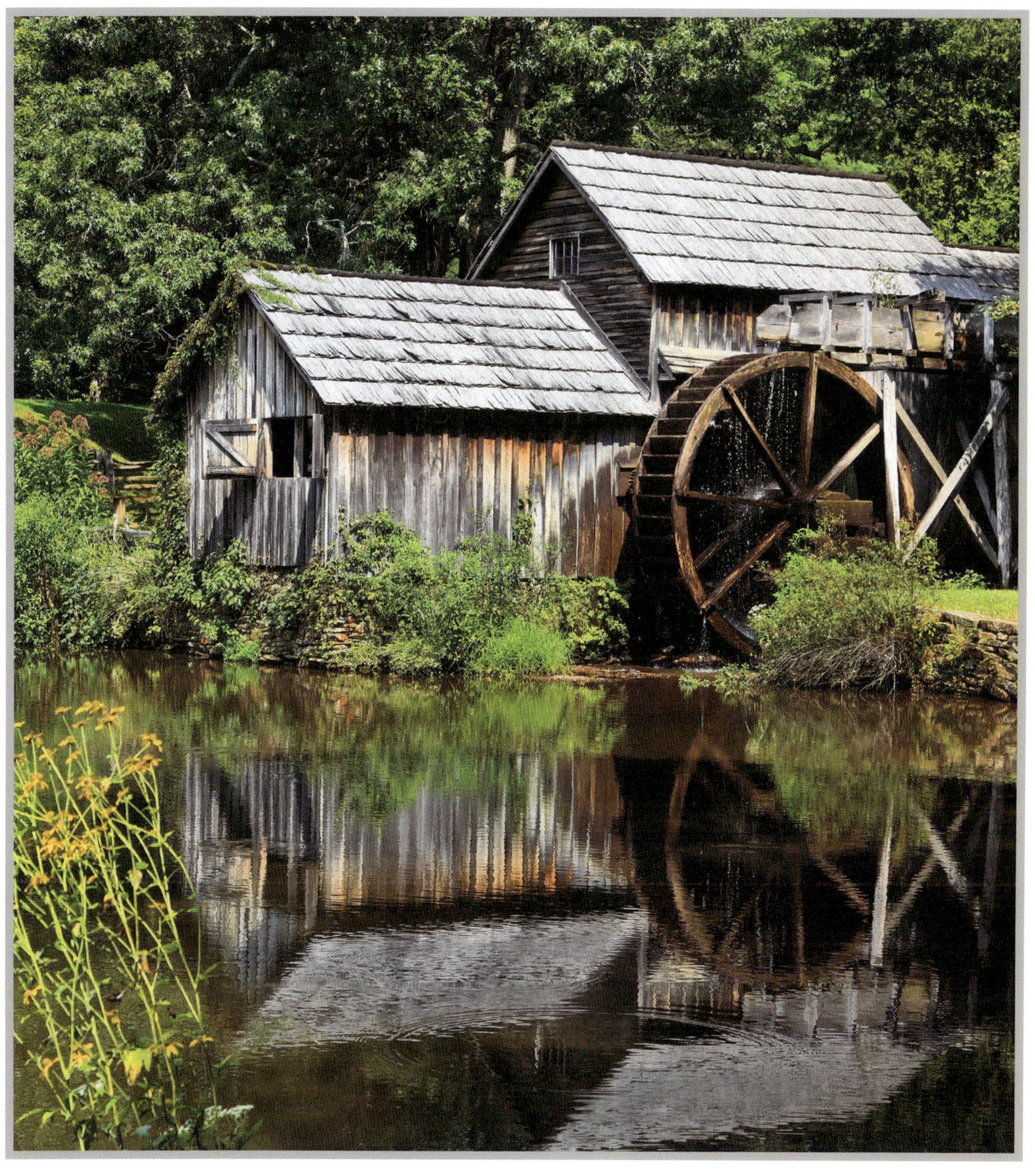

As calm as a millpond.

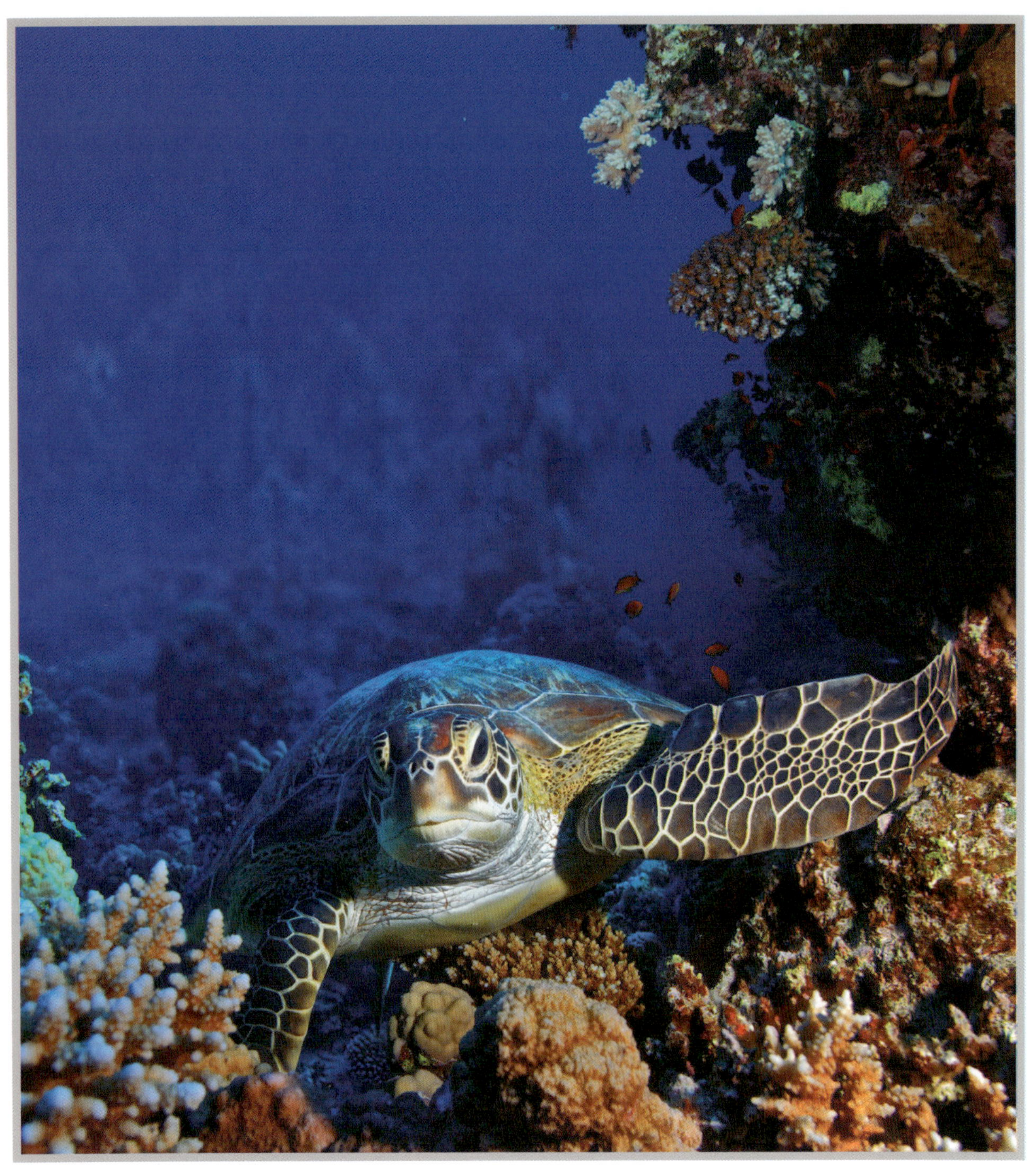

As deep as the ocean.

Quick Quiz 4: Strange expressions

1 As tough as old _ _ _ _ _ _ .

2 As fit as a _ _ _ _ _ _ _ .

3 As scarce as hen's _ _ _ _ _ _ .

4 As boring as watching paint _ _ _ .

5 As plain as the nose on your _ _ _ _ .

6 As happy as a pig in _ _ _ .

7 As snug as a bug in a _ _ _ .

Answers coming up!

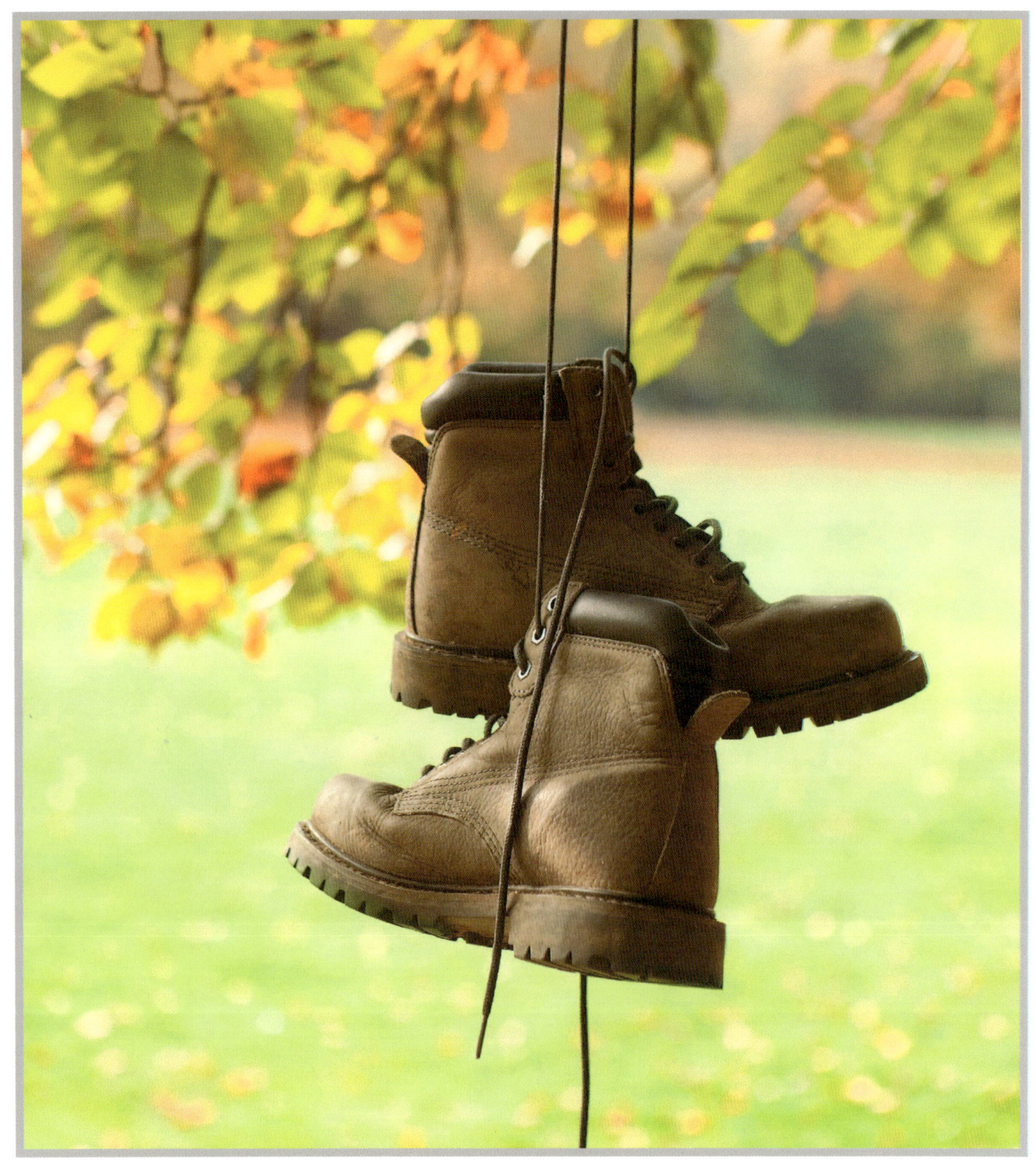

As tough as old boots.

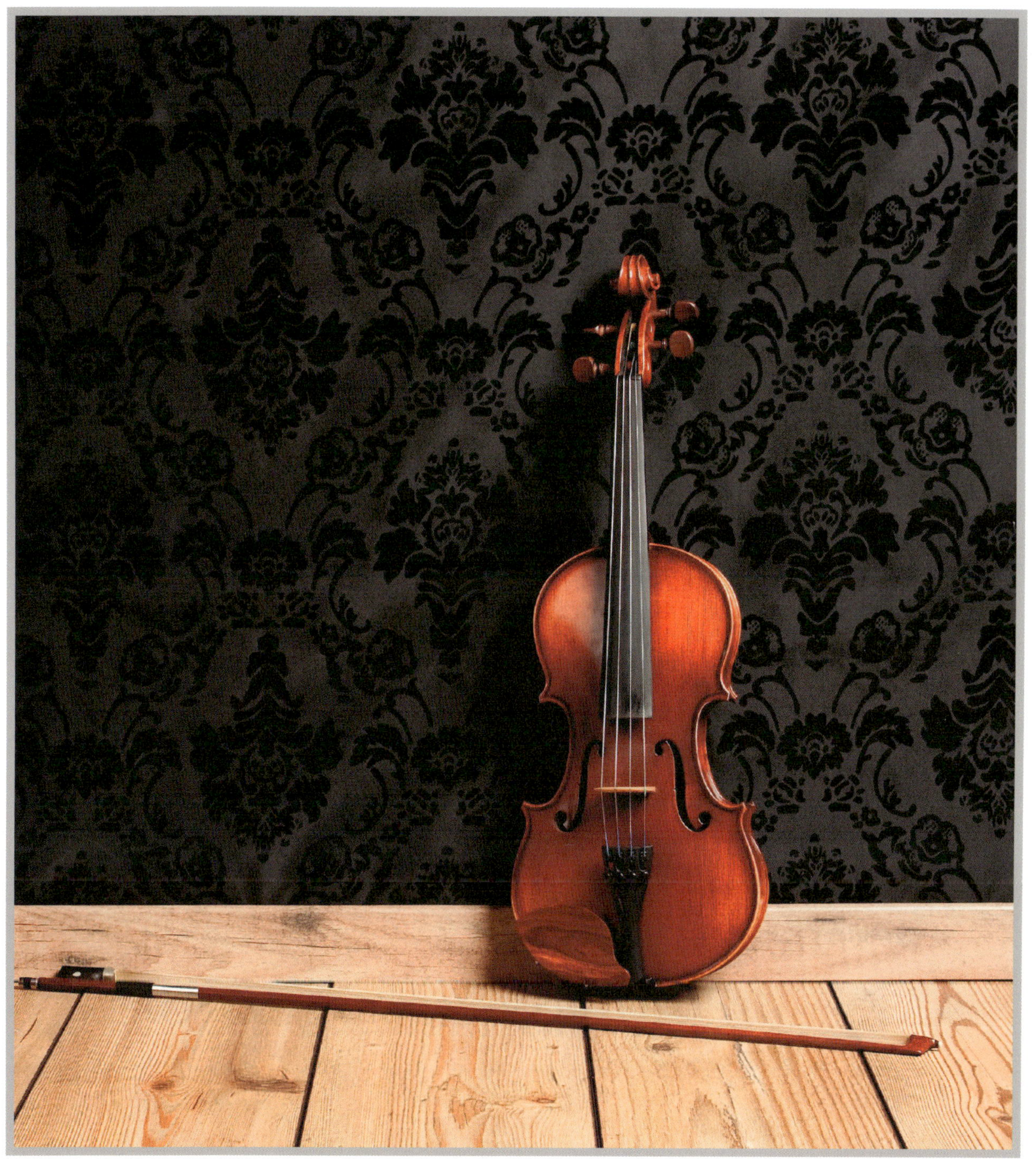

As fit as a fiddle.

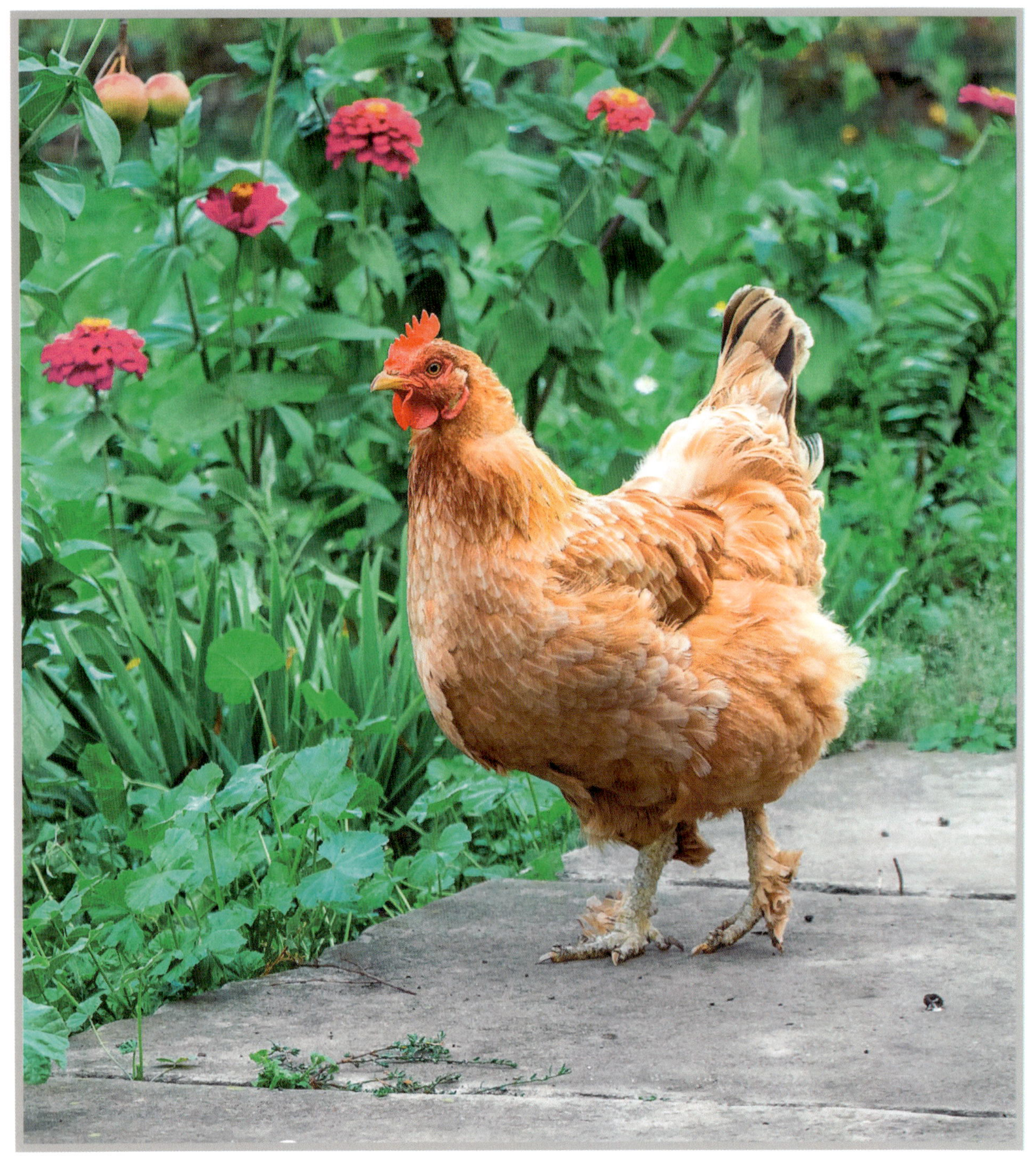

As scarce as hen's teeth.

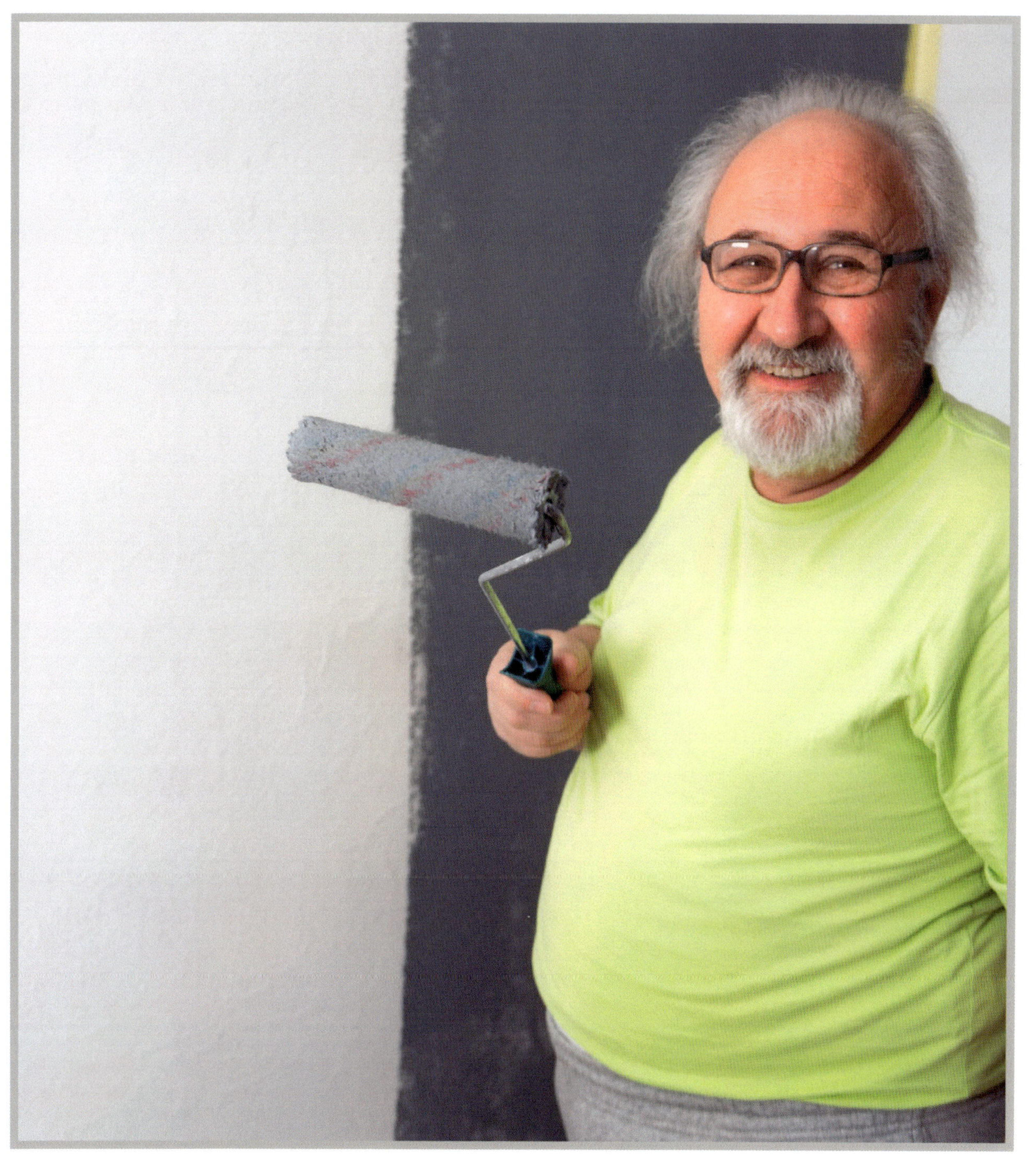

As boring as watching paint dry.

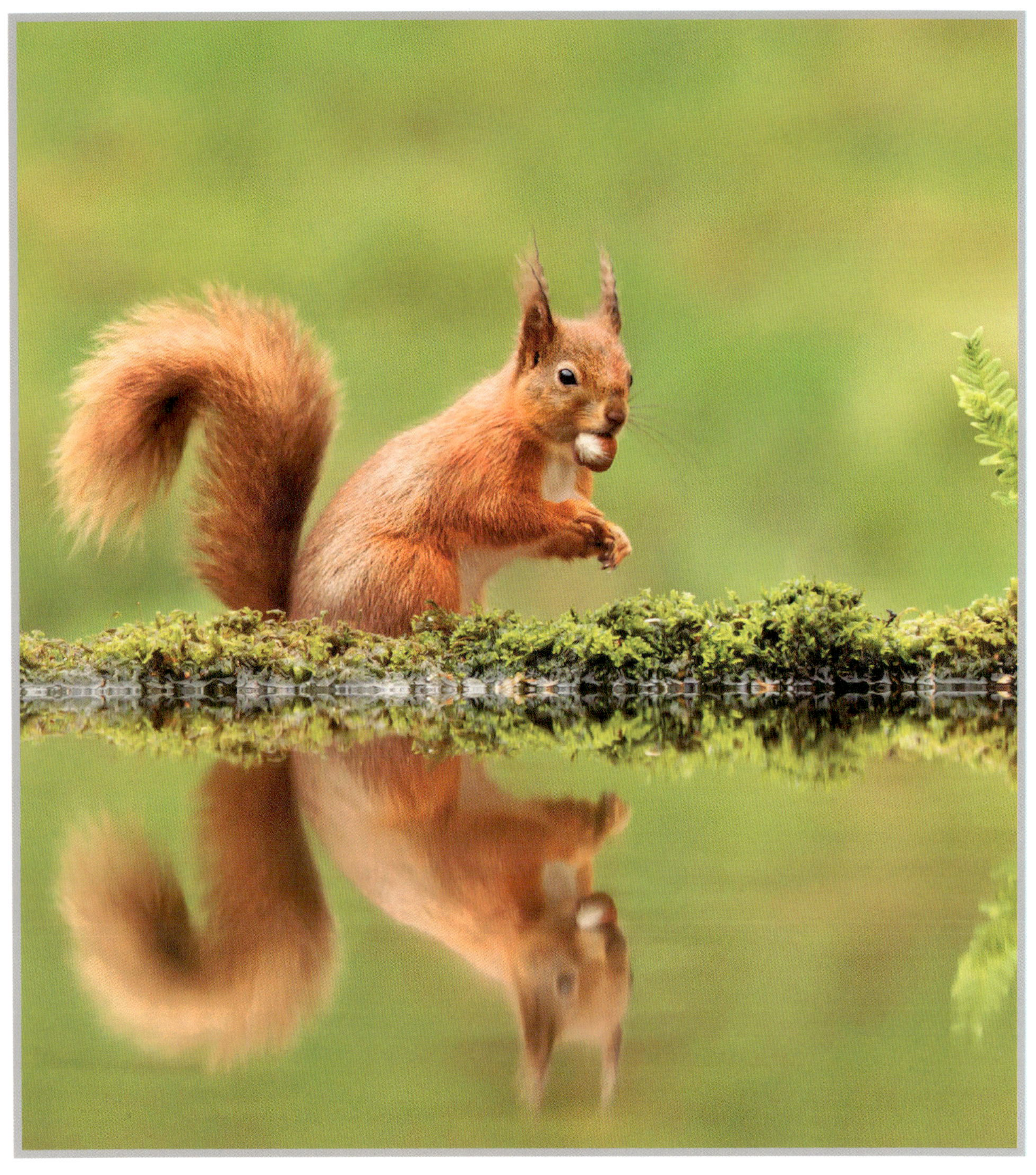

As plain as the nose on your face.

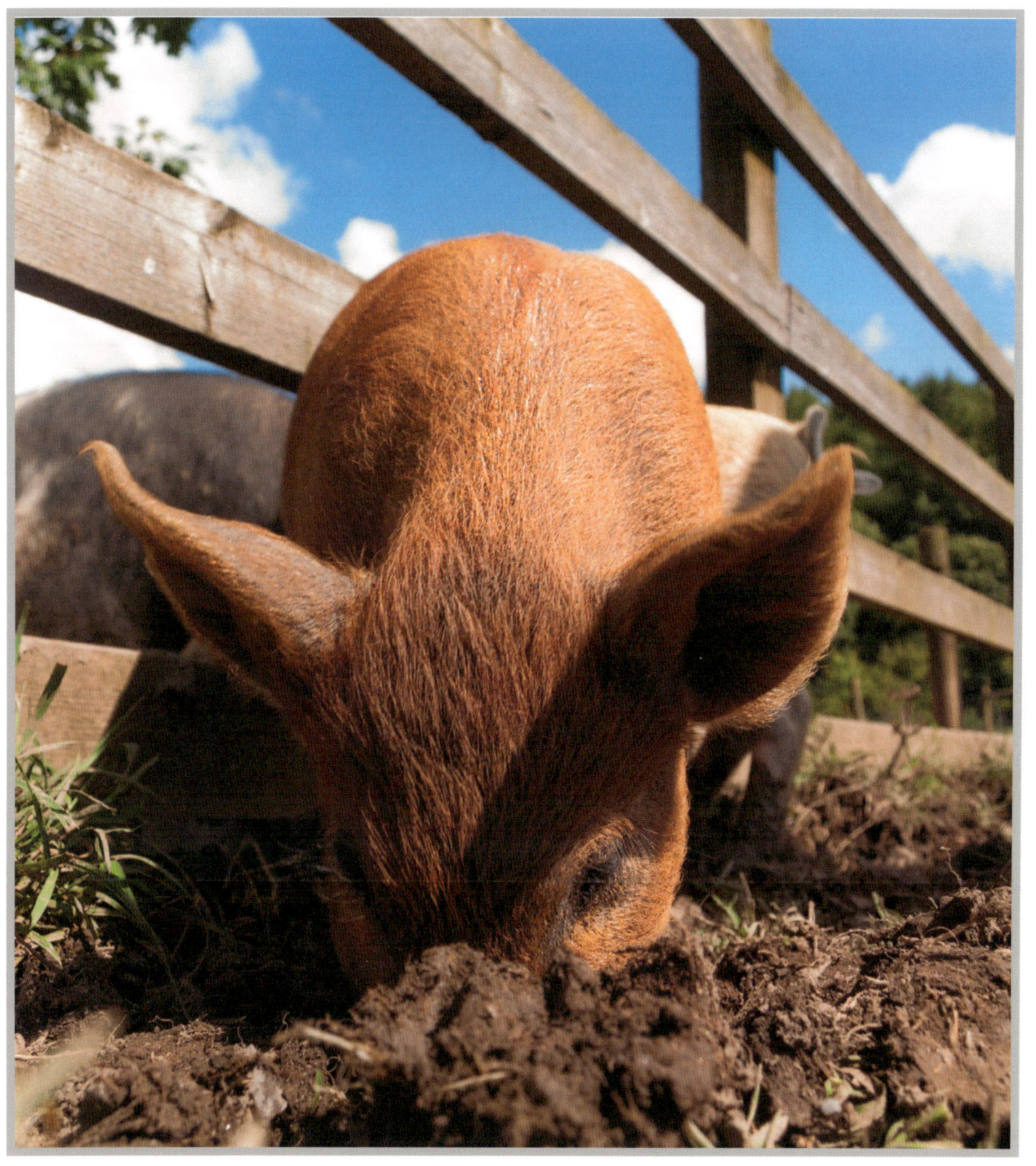

As happy as a pig in mud.

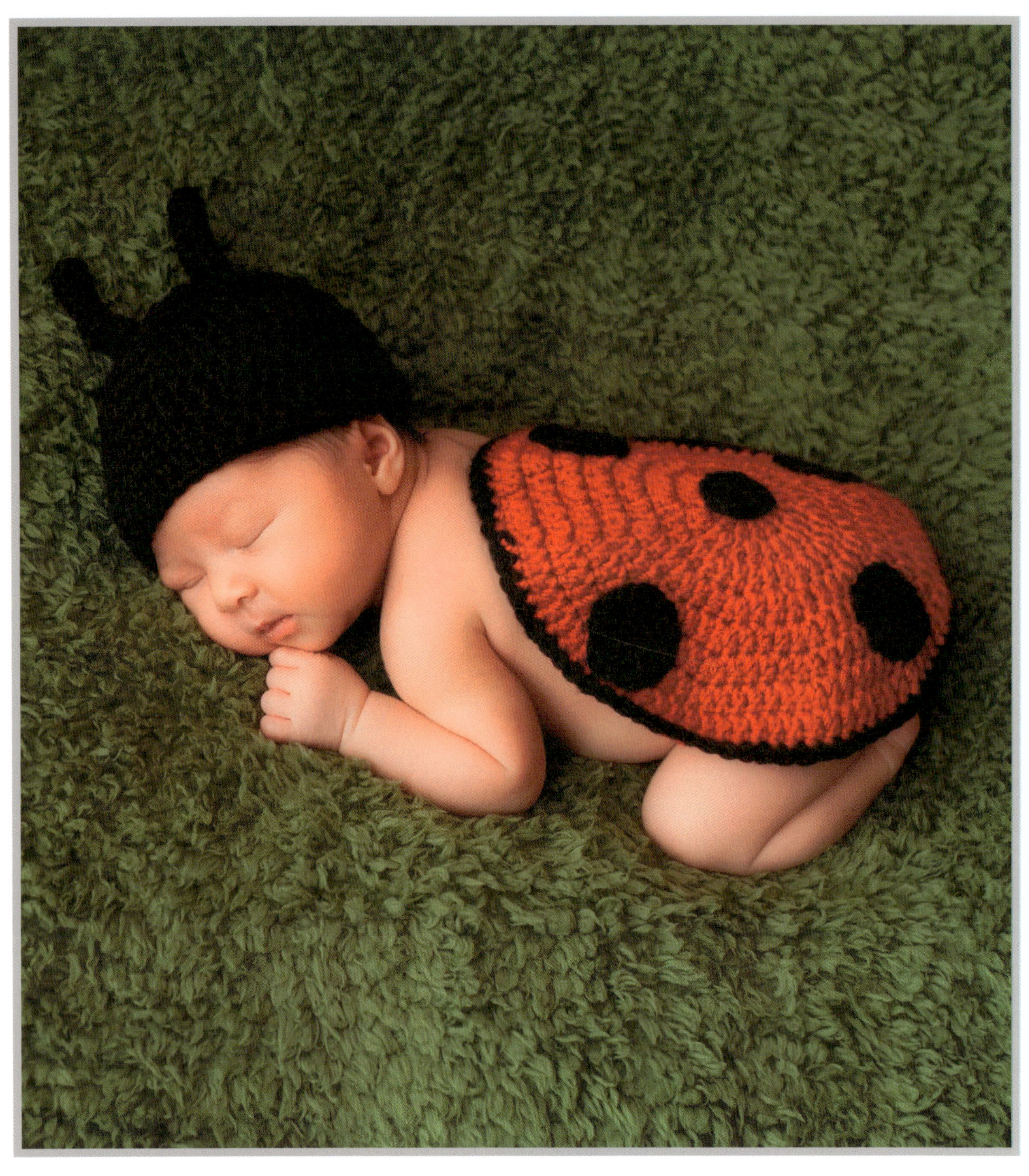

As snug as a bug in a rug.

Congratulations,
but it's not quite the end...

Here are a few bonus questions.

1 **Do you sleep like a _ _ _ ?**

2 **Can you swim like a _ _ _ _ ?**

3 **Do you eat like a _ _ _ _ _ ?**

4 **Do you smell like a _ _ _ _ ?**

Answers coming up!

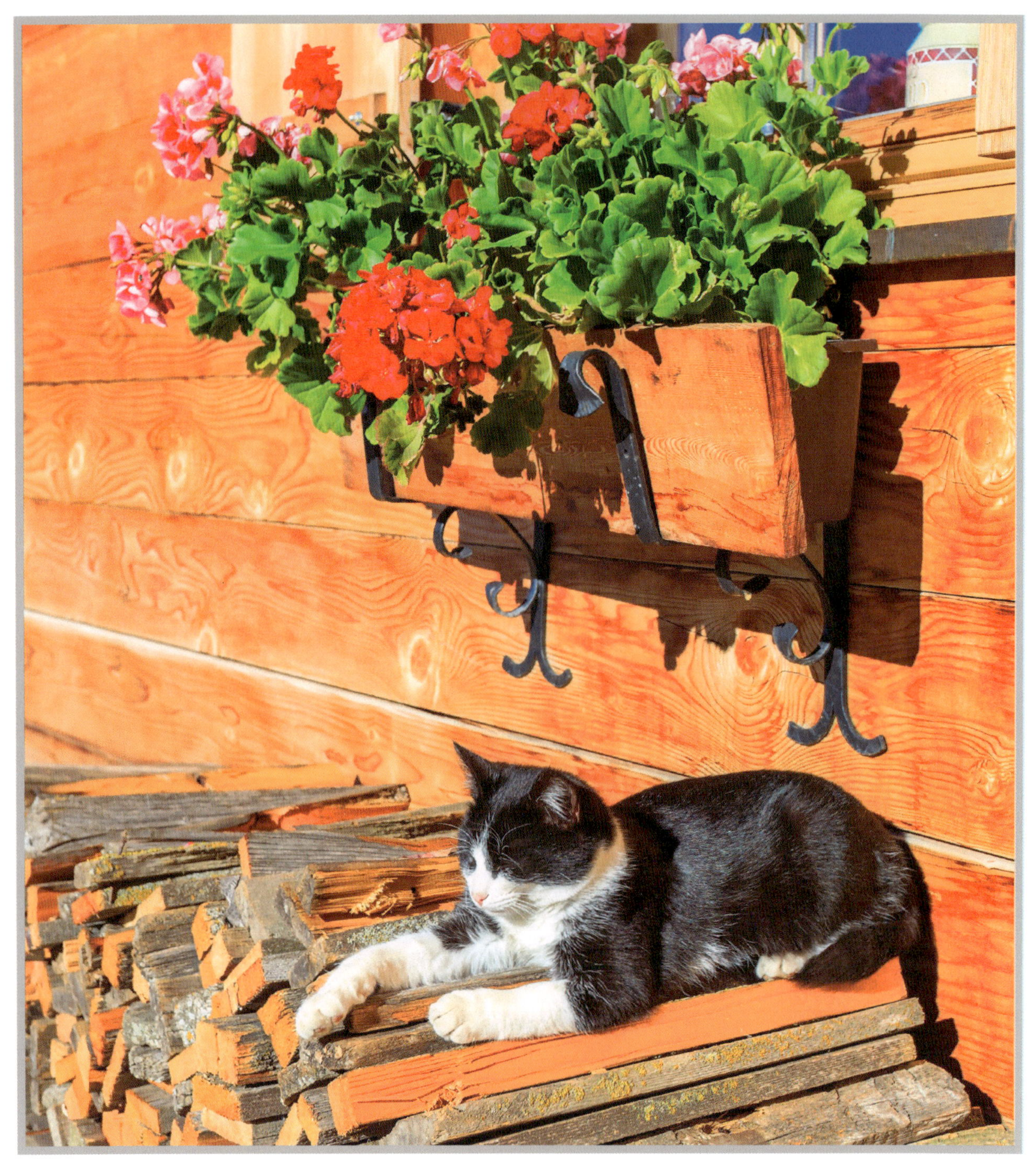

Do you sleep like a log?

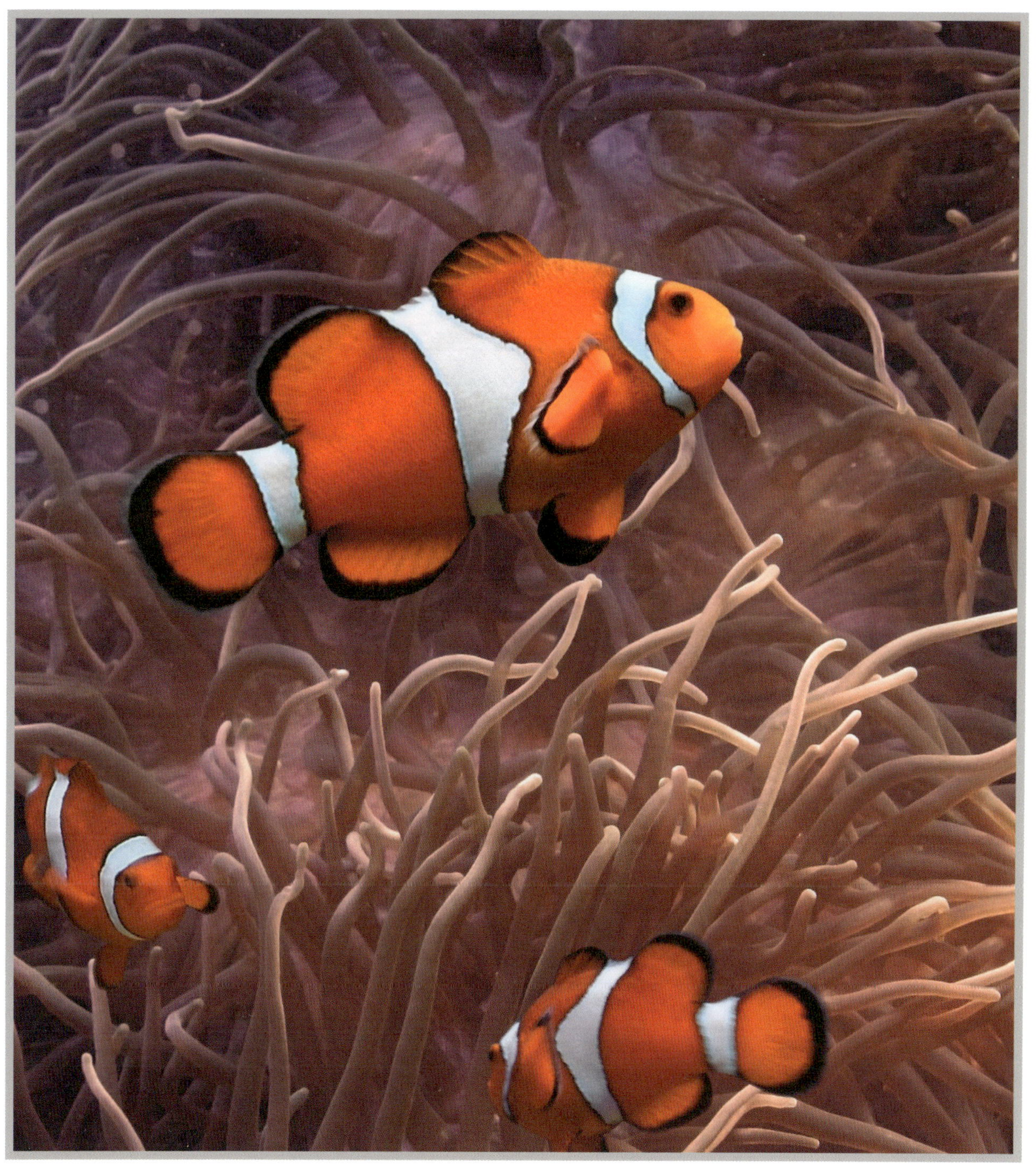

Can you swim like a fish?

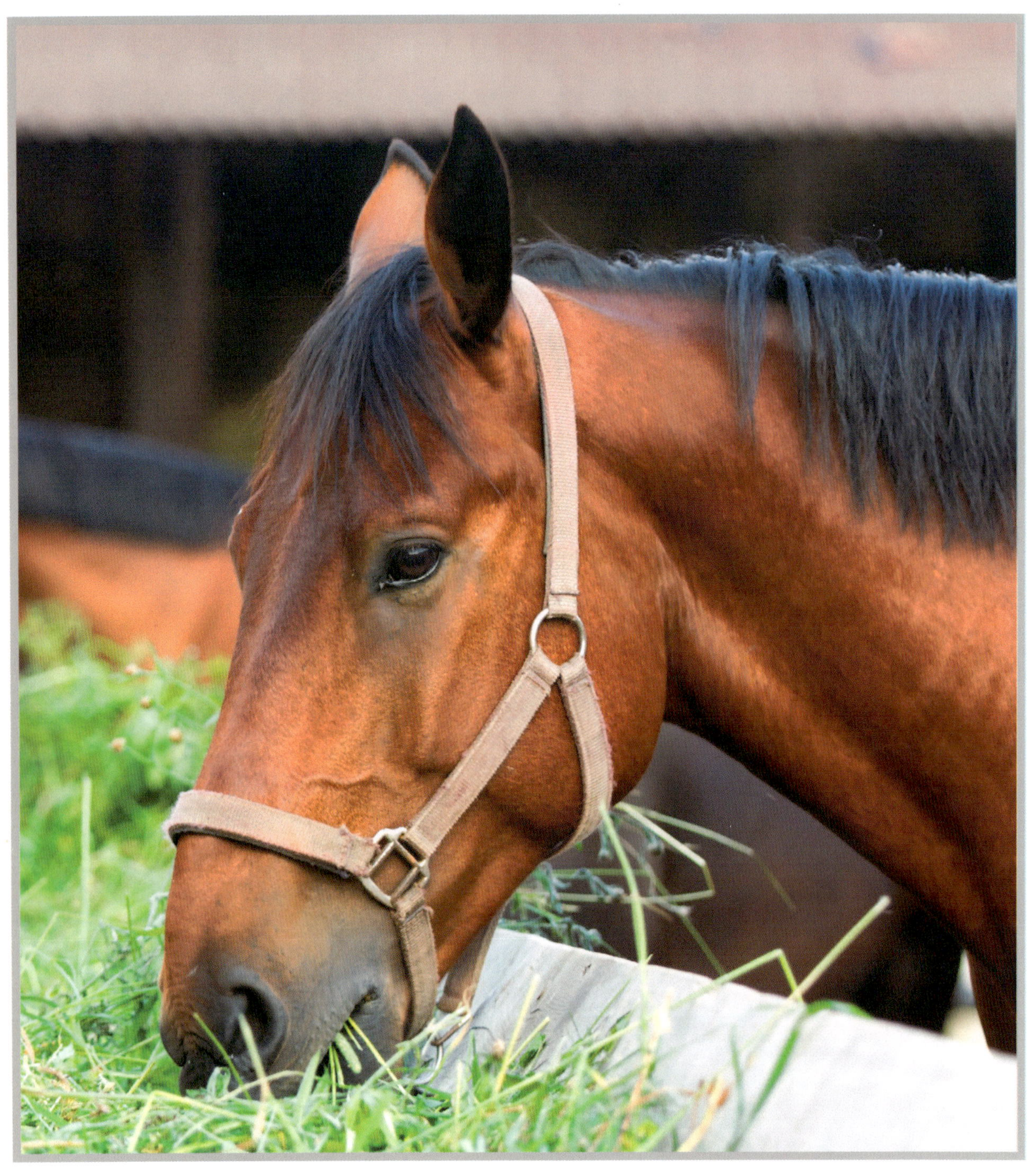

Do you eat like a horse?

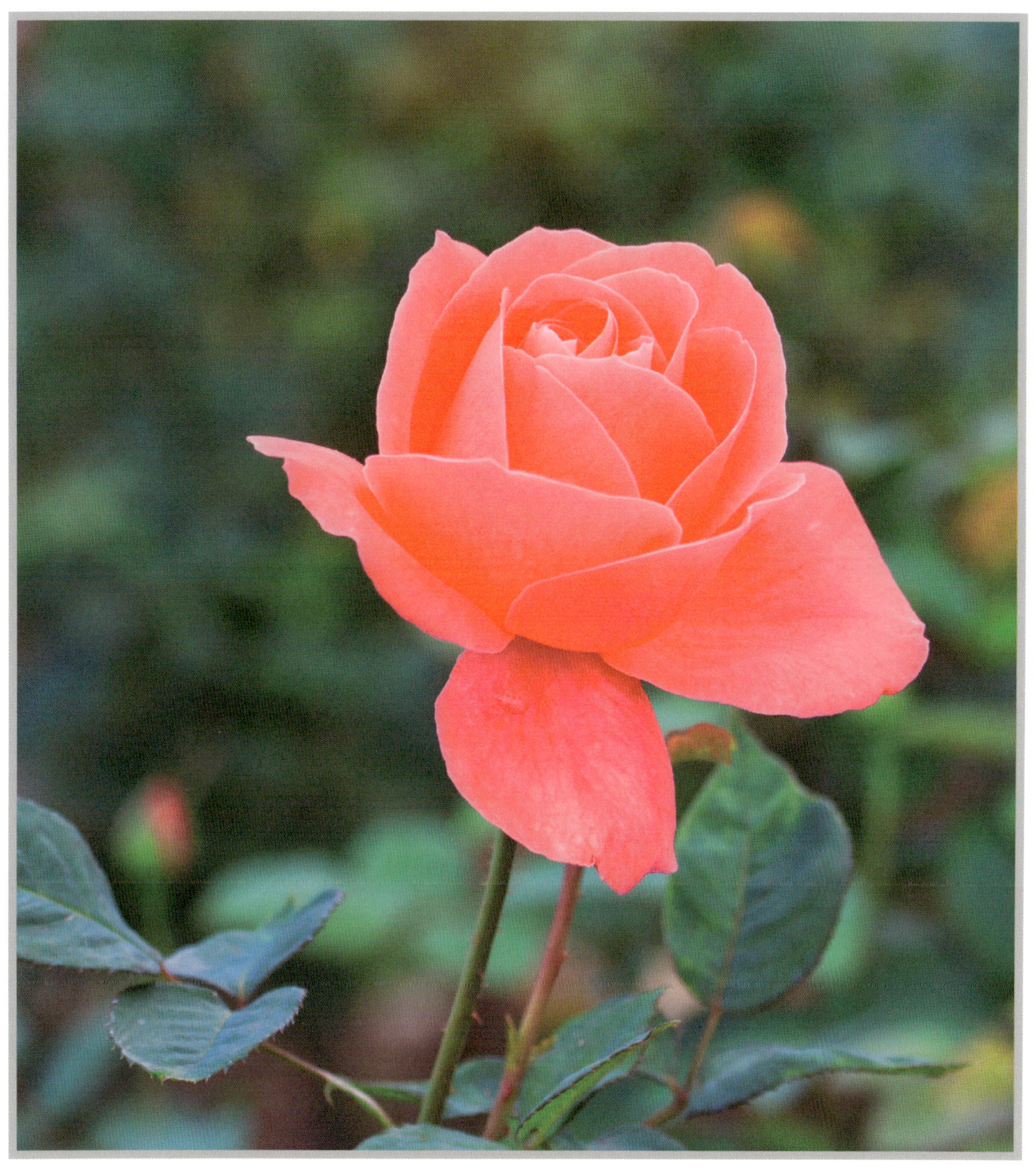

Do you smell like a rose?

Thanks for reading!
Did you enjoy this book?
There are more in the series!

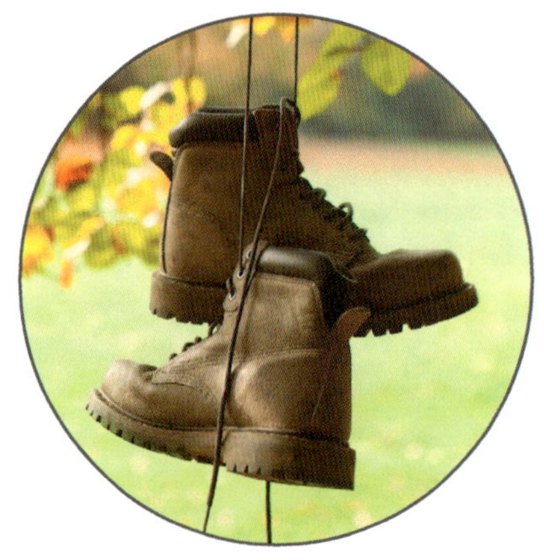

This collection of traditional sayings and photos
selected by © Unforgettable Notes 2022
thebooknextdoor.com/unforgettablenotes
Series: Illustrated Traditional Sayings

The usual copyright rules apply.
These traditional sayings are in the Public Domain.

Printed in Great Britain
by Amazon

31936934R00025